Essential Midwifery Practice:
Postnatal Care

Essential Midwifery Practice: Postnatal Care

Edited by

Sheena Byrom
RGN, RM, MA

Grace Edwards
RGN, RM, ADM, Cert Ed, Med, PhD

Debra Bick
RM, BA, MMedSc, PhD

⟨W⟩WILEY-BLACKWELL

A John Wiley & Sons, Ltd., Publication

Library of Congress Cataloging-in-Publication Data
Essential midwifery practice. Postnatal care / edited by Sheena Byrom, Grace Edwards, Debra Bick.
p. ; cm.
Includes bibliographical references and index.
ISBN 978-1-4051-7091-8 (pbk. : alk. paper)
1. Postnatal care. 2. Midwifery. I. Byrom, Sheena. II. Edwards, Grace, RN. III. Bick, Debra. IV. Title: Postnatal care.
[DNLM: 1. Postnatal Care. 2. Maternal Welfare. 3. Midwifery. WQ 500 E78 2010]
RG801.E87 2010
618.6 – dc22
2009020249

A catalogue record for this book is available from the British Library.

Set in 10/12.5pt Palatino by Laserwords Private Limited, Chennai, India
Printed in Singapore by Ho Printing Singapore Pte Ltd

1   2010

Contents

Foreword

The care of a woman and her baby in the immediate hours, days and weeks following birth can make an enormous difference to their long-term health and well-being. The content and timing of postnatal care led by midwives was formalised in the United Kingdom following a statutory legislation that was first introduced in England in 1902. Then there were concerns that too many women were dying following birth. The provision of midwifery care for all women including postnatal contacts in hospital and in the home, together with improved public health and advances in medicine, led to a dramatic fall in the UK maternal mortality rate. Sadly, the main causes of death at the beginning of the twentieth century in the United Kingdom, haemorrhage and sepsis, continue to kill hundreds of thousands of women globally. Postnatal care has frequently been portrayed as the 'Cinderella' of the maternity service, and often appears to be the least important and resourced part of the woman's journey through pregnancy and birth.

In the United Kingdom, the last decade has witnessed a decline in the provision of midwifery postnatal care contacts; conversely evidence of the potential benefits of effective postnatal care for maternal health has been published. The increasing 'invisibility' of postnatal care is an issue that should concern all who recognise the importance of good maternal health not only for the well-being of a family but also for the well-being of wider society. Postnatal services have been affected by a shortage of midwifery staff and increased pressure on our units as a result of the increasing birth rate. We also know that women may be entering pregnancy in poorer health, which in turn has implications for the level of care they require during and after they have given birth. It is within this current context of care that this book has been written. It will be an extremely valuable asset for those who wish to understand why postnatal care is an invaluable component of good public health and how the planning and content of care could make a difference to all women and in particular to the most vulnerable women and families in our society. The authors of each chapter are all acknowledged experts in their field. Many are also midwives in practice and as such not only are they aware of the pressures on postnatal services but they also offer insights into how current resources could be used more effectively. I hope that by reading the book you will also view the need to accord equal priority to the planning and provision of postnatal care, as with all other aspects of pregnancy and birth care. For many women, the postnatal period is the time when they feel most vulnerable, and sadly it is also the time when they feel most neglected by the health services. This book will make a tremendous contribution to understanding the public health consequences of effective postnatal care and why it should not persist as the 'poor relation' of our maternity services.

Cathy Warwick
General Secretary of the Royal College of Midwives, UK

Preface

Sally Marchant's chapter examines how the status of midwifery and the role of postnatal care evolved, mainly within the context of maternity service provision in the United Kingdom. The relationship between the health and the well-being of a woman and the care received after giving birth are addressed in terms of major maternal morbidity, for example, post-partum haemorrhage. In ancient Egyptian and Roman societies, historical sources describe the role of the midwife and some of the herbs and other preparations used in their practice. Centuries later, the Catholic Church in mainland Europe evolved to become the dominant power in society, with powers to license midwifery practice, wherein midwives were required to take an oath promising that 'magic' would not be used in their practice. Traditional customs and rituals related to care after giving birth, highlighting the fear of death from sepsis or haemorrhage, were incorporated into religious and social frameworks, many of which persist in some cultures to the present day. Towards the beginning of the twentieth century, when acknowledgement in the United Kingdom that public health initiatives were essential if the population's health were to improve, a raft of measures were introduced including the first Midwives Act in England, which paved the way for the supervision and regulation of midwifery practice and training. The implications of the Midwives Act for women's health, midwifery practice and subsequent impact on the timing and content of postnatal care are outlined.

Debra Bick's chapter on issues relating to the current provision of postnatal care outlines as to why during the transition to the twenty-first century, changes in public health priorities and acknowledgement that traditional midwifery models were not meeting maternal needs led to calls to revise postnatal care. For the first time, evidence was available that clearly showed that many women experienced long-term physical and psychological problems after giving birth. Minimal guidance for midwives on the content and timing of care, which had altered little during the course of the previous century, resulted in a system that did not identify or meet women's needs. Despite evidence that revising midwifery care could make a difference to aspects of women's health, pressure on maternity services continues to impact on resources for postnatal care, with a seemingly low priority placed on provision of care planned and tailored to individual needs. Ironically, this is against a background of policy publications that have acknowledged the potential benefit of postnatal care for public health. In developing countries where thousands of women continue to die each year as a consequence of post-partum haemorrhage, the need to view postnatal care as part of a continuum of care for Safe Motherhood has been highlighted. Although maternal health needs differ greatly across the globe, effective postnatal care could make an enormous difference to the lives of all women and their babies. The challenge of how to ensure that this is implemented remains.

Jane Yelland's focuses on the provision of postnatal care in Chapter 3, within the first 1 to 2 weeks of birth from the perspective of service users (the woman) and providers (the midwives). This is an area with a limited but developing evidence base. Most work to date has been conducted in Western countries, where surveys have highlighted women's concerns with aspects of their postnatal care, particularly hospital-based care. Despite differences in maternity care models internationally, women report similar experiences and views, which are outlined in the chapter within the context of the diversity of models of care and care providers. There is increasing interest in eliciting the views of service users; however, this is raising issues of how to define and objectively measure outcomes such as satisfaction with care. A range of approaches used in research studies to examine experiences are outlined, as are consequences for validity and generalisability of study findings. Evidence of the impact of revisions to maternity care on women's experiences and views is described, with domains and factors that impact care perceptions presented under four broad themes. There has been a dearth of research into the views of midwives who provide postnatal care; nevertheless, publications to date highlight a range of resource constraints perceived as impacting the ability to provide care based on need.

The emotions of becoming a mother are explored in Chapter 4, and Kathryn Gutteridge provides an insight into the psychological impact of motherhood on women. The chapter provides insights into the effects of pregnancy and birth on parenting and nurture instincts, and describes other influences both social and medical, that impact on the mother–infant dyad. The pressures of modern society and unrealistic expectations also play a part in the mother's psyche, and perinatal mental health is influenced adversely by these factors. The author highlights how pregnancy has become the business of others, instead of just the mothers, and suggests that this may undermine the woman's perceptions of her own capability to give birth to or parent her baby. The role of the midwife is a crucial part of this process and can positively or negatively influence the health and well-being of both mother and baby.

Involving service users in the NHS has been very much driven by the health and social care policy, increasingly so in the past 10 years. Sheena Byrom and Anna Gaudion describe the importance of involving women and their families in the planning and delivery of maternity services in Chapter 5, both from the perspective of the organisation and department, and more importantly, the benefits of the individual involved. Community engagement models are described, and examples of positive collaboration between service users and maternity services highlight the potential impact for local communities. There is a suggestion that the empowering model of woman- centred care can positively influence not only the impact of the birth process but also the woman's life thereafter.

Chapter 6 focuses on morbidity in the postnatal period and its impact, and Christine McCourt and Maria Helena Bastos argue that it is very common for women to experience a number of postnatal health problems. They propose that it is important that women understand that some of their experiences are 'normal'. The authors warn that the impact of morbidity on women's well-being needs to be taken seriously by midwives and other healthcare professionals, with sufficient, appropriate support and information offered to women. postnatal morbidity, both physical and psychological, may have major long-term impacts on maternal and infant health. While this is challenging, particularly for hard-pressed staff in busy health services, it also forms an important opportunity for midwives and other healthcare providers to make a positive difference to public health at a key point of transition. Midwives may make a difference to health both by preventing morbidity and by responding effectively to the problems that women do experience.

Implementing UNICEF's Baby Friendly Hospital Initiative is described by Val Finigan as being a positive and successful approach to improve breastfeeding rates. The chapter provides the reader with an insight into the benefits of adapting and achieving the standards of the BFHI in practice and the details involved when embarking on the programme. The benefits of breastfeeding for mother and infant are reinforced, together with essential evidence relating to health inequalities, and the consequential importance for promoting and supporting breastfeeding strategies for success.

In Chapter 8, Anita Fleming and Jill Cooper detail the importance of providing extra support in the postnatal period to the woman who is vulnerable, whatever the reason. The impact of vulnerability is double edged, as both mother and infant are potentially at risk, and intensive support is suggested to maximise opportunity for improved health outcomes. The authors suggest support should begin in the antenatal period, with the mobilisation of support networks to assist when the baby is born. Various strategies and good practice examples are detailed, providing the reader with ideas from their own practice.

Selina Nylander and Christine Shea share their thoughts about working in partnership, and therefore building on the previous chapter to enhance knowledge for supporting families in their parenting journey. They describe how health professionals may work in partnership using the guidance of the Child Health Promotion Programme. The issue of fragmented care is discussed, particularly around support for the continuation of breastfeeding and including partners in postnatal care. Government policy is used to support choice for women and their families and midwives are introduced to the commissioning cycle. Finally, engagement of Practice-Based Commissioning and the third sector are explored and ways in which midwives may engage are suggested.

New parents rarely understand how having a child can change life and all parents seek reassurance that their infant is healthy and developing as expected. Annie Dixon describes how the transition to parenthood can be stressful, and how midwives can positively influence this rite of passage. She explores the meaning of family and explains how this may mean different things to different people and highlights how personal beliefs and cultures will affect parenting. She discusses positive parenting and points out ways in which parents may be supported and empowered through non-judgemental support. Finally, she describes how parents may be empowered, using the early examination of the newborn as an example of working with parents.

Sexual health is a major concern within public health and is a key driver for the Government's White Paper – *Choosing Health*. The postnatal period is the ideal time to address issues around sexual health and ensure that the woman and her partner are well informed about prevention of infection, family planning and risk taking. Grace Edwards and Susie Gardiner describe the historical trends in sexual health and the recent trends in sexual activity, particularly amongst young people. The commonest sexually transmitted infections are explained and the current prevalence, consequences and treatment are explored. The psychology of attitudes around sexual health and behaviour and advice for midwives on offering support and sign posting for encouraging a healthy approach to sexual health, particularly in the postnatal period, is discussed.

Notes on the Contributors

Maria Helena Bastos is a research associate at King's College, London, and teaching assistant in Midwifery and Women's Health at Thames Valley University. She is currently conducting research towards a PhD. Maria Helena trained as a gynaecologist and obstetrician, and practised for almost 20 years, in addition to lecturing in Brazil. Having worked as a programme officer of REHUNA (Brazilian Network for Humanisation of Birth), she gained experience promoting evidence-based childbirth practices in her country. As a founding member of Brazil's National Association of Doulas (ANDO) – supporting the development and implementation of educational programmes for doula support in public maternity hospitals in Brazil – she gained skills coordinating community-based programmes in diverse communities in Rio de Janeiro and Brasilia.

Currently, Maria Helena works as a part-time research associate in a UK Department of Health funded project at King's College London, developing and implementing a training package for maternity staff to support women and their birth partners to have a positive labour and birth experience.

Debra Bick was professor of midwifery at Thames Valley University before being appointed to King's College and had previously worked at the Royal College of Nursing, where she headed a national guideline development programme, and the University of Birmingham where she worked on several large randomised controlled trials (RCTs) to examine the impact of interventions during and after birth on maternal, physical and psychological morbidity.

Debra's research interests include postnatal health, the organisation of maternity services and approaches to evidence synthesis and transfer to enhance maternal and infant health. She has published numerous papers, commentaries and book chapters around these issues and has edited several books. She was a member of the postnatal subgroup of the NSF for Children, Young People and Maternity Services (DoH 2004) and Clinical Advisor on the NICE postnatal care guideline (NICE 2006).

Debra is editor-in-chief of *Midwifery: An International Journal*, an international editorial board member of several journals, visiting professor at the University of Sao Paulo and Bournemouth University and was visiting fellow at the Women's and Children's Hospital in Adelaide in July 2008.

Current research projects include the Hospital to Home postnatal care study and a UK-wide matched pair cluster RCT of a training intervention to enhance midwifery and obstetric management of perineal trauma. Debra is co-investigator on an NIHR RfPB funded trial of diamorphine compared with pethidine for pain relief during labour and an NIHR HTA funded trial of upright and supine positions in labour among primiparous women who have epidural analgesia. She was a co-investigator on two recently completed NIHR SDO projects. One project assessed the impact of use of protocols and care pathways to support the use of evidence in practice and the second project assessed their impact on clinical decision making.

Sheena Byrom has been working as a midwife since 1978, in hospital and community settings. Sheena worked for 10 years in a maternity home (birth centre) and believes her midwifery philosophy and expertise was positively influenced during this time. Sheena has managerial experience and is a supervisor of midwives.

Sheena currently works as a consultant midwife in public health, a post that is a joint appointment between the University of Central Lancashire and East Lancashire Hospitals NHS Trust. At the University, she contributes to the research agenda and assists in developing links between academia and practice. Sheena was nominated twice to meet the Prime Minister for NHS services to the community, invited as a member of the Secretary of State for Health's Clinical Sounding Board in 2007 and regularly participates in midwifery matters at the Department of Health. Sheena was a member of the Postnatal Care NICE clinical guideline development group for England and Wales. Other interests include leadership philosophy, promotion of normal birth, community development and health inequalities.

Jill Cooper works as a caseload midwife at East Lancashire Hospitals Trust, providing one-to-one care to vulnerable women and families. She qualified as a midwife in 2002 and has worked within East Lancashire Hospitals Trust since that time as a rotational midwife, a team midwife and more latterly as a caseload midwife. Jill firmly believes that all women need to be placed at the centre of their care, no matter how complex their case, in order to promote a positive experience during their pregnancy, labour, birth and early parenting.

Annie Dixon qualified as a general and sick children's nurse in 1986. She has gained over 20 years experience in a variety of settings including regional neonatal units, district general hospitals and community and higher education whilst working with infants and their families. She has a PG Cert in health service management, a Certificate in counselling and R23 Enhanced Neonatal Practice, all of which helped her to successfully complete an MSc by research exploring communication between parents and nurses. Annie's wider research interests include communicating with parents, family- centred care, shared decision-making, clinical supervision, training and education.

Grace Edwards qualified as a midwife in 1978 working as a hospital midwife and a community midwife for 12 years, during which time she completed the advanced diploma of midwifery and the certificate in education. She worked as a midwife teacher in 1988 and completed a Masters in Education. In 1993, she took up post as regional co-ordinator for CESDI (the Confidential Enquiry into Stillbirths and Deaths in Infancy) and the Congenital Anomaly Survey, a post she held until 2002. During this time, she completed a PhD in people's perceptions of healthy pregnancy. Since 2002, she has been employed as consultant midwife in public health in Liverpool. In 2004, she accepted a post as principal lecturer in midwifery research at the University of Central Lancashire, a post she held until 2007. In 2005, she was appointed as national midwifery assessor for the Confidential Enquiry into Maternal and Child health for maternal mortality.

Val Finigan MBE is the infant feeding coordinator for Pennine Acute NHS Trust. Her core role is to implement the UNICEF Baby Friendly Initiative standards across the four hospitals that make up the trust and to encourage uptake of BFHI within the four surrounding PCTs. Val has worked in the NHS for 30 years and she is committed to improving the support and care offered to women and their families. Val is a doctoral student with the University of Salford and her studies are focused on women's experience of skin-to-skin contact. Val has published in peer-reviewed journals and published a book.

Anita Fleming works at East Lancashire Hospitals Trust, leading a team of midwives providing a caseload model of care to women from vulnerable groups. Since qualifying as a midwife 19 years ago, Anita has gained substantial all-round midwifery experience, having worked in all departments of the hospital prior to becoming an integrated team midwife, and later team leader on the same team. This was followed by working in the role of Sure Start midwife before taking up her present role 5 years ago. Anita is passionate about promoting normality in childbirth, and more importantly, in promoting positive birth experiences for the most vulnerable maternity service users.

Susie Gardiner began working for Wirral Brook (a young person's sexual health service) as outreach co-ordinator in 1997, combining this with working as a senior officer for supported housing. In 2002, she was appointed as teenage pregnancy co-ordinator for Knowsley PCT and later went on to become commissioning and modernisation manager for public health in the Borough, with a remit for sexual health. Alongside this, she completed an MSc in public health. Susie is now employed by Liverpool PCT as senior practitioner for public health improvement and is public health lead for sexual health. She is currently undertaking a postgraduate certificate in leadership and supports trainees in health needs assessment and public health for the RCOG and faculty of sexual and reproductive health care's subspecialty training in sexual and reproductive health.

Anna Gaudion has an academic background in anthropology, museum ethnography/anthropology of art and refugee studies. She has an eclectic career pathway that weaves through the arts and maternity services, working in the weekend as a midwife on the 'Bank' at Guys and St Thomas' NHS Trust during her studies and career as a curator in the ethnographic department of the British Museum, arts critic and lecturer in the anthropological aspects of women's health at Kings College. In 2004, she directed and made the film *Florence, the experience in becoming a mother in exile*. More recently, she has gained experience in accessing and consulting vulnerable groups about maternity services; a Health Equity Audit of access to maternity services in SE London (Maternity Matters Early Adopter site) and a Needs Assessments concerning the specific needs of asylum seekers and refugees (Brunel University). As part of the Polyanna Project, she has ongoing experience and learning by working in consultation with women, their partners and families to produce picture-based information resources, the process and findings of which are recorded in a visual diary and report as a means for users of the service to have a voice. She is currently the project lead for the Centering Pregnancy Pilot at Kings College Hospital, London.

Kathryn Gutteridge began her career in the 1970s in nursing. However, midwifery was always her ambition and particularly the nurturance of midwifery-led care. She spent 11 years as a community midwife where she felt completely at home with both the environment and the nature of the work. Following this, she began work as a consultant midwife, formerly employed at University Hospital of Leicester for 4 years but more recently at Sandwell & West Birmingham NHS Trust.

Kathryn is a practising psychotherapist interested in the emotional impact of childbirth, in part because of her own mothering experiences and research. Working closely for many years raising awareness around the issues of maternal mental health and supporting both women and all those who work in maternity care situations, she has engaged directly with women to understand this phenomenon and researched emotional transition to motherhood, gaining an MSc in counselling and psychotherapy.

Raising awareness for maternal mental health, and particularly women surviving sexual abuse, she co-founded Sanctum Midwives, campaigning on maternity care and sexual abuse. This is a poorly understood area of maternity care and she believes both as a professional and as a survivor herself that it is vital to ensure a positive birth and mothering experience. Kathryn believes that positive mental health is the cornerstone to mothering and self-fulfilment.

First and foremost, she is a mother, wife and latterly grandmother: her personal life has always largely informed her practice and she is always careful to remember that the women she meets are also like her in that they belong to a family.

Sally Marchant trained as a midwife in Scotland and spent the following 10 years mainly caring for postnatal women in her local maternity unit. An interest in industrial relations led to a period working for the Royal College of Midwives and from there, to the National Perinatal Epidemiology Unit in Oxford. This laid the foundations for work on a number of research projects and then a move to involvement in pre- and post-registration education at Bournemouth University until she became the editor for the *MIDIRS Midwifery Digest*, a post she has held for the last 6 years. Throughout this time, postnatal care has been her main interest and was the focus for her PhD looking at the role of midwives in the postnatal assessment of uterine involution. As part of her PhD work, she also became interested in aspects of midwifery history that led to many forages in the dusty attics and cellars of bookshops up and down the country, resulting in a small but interesting collection of textbooks and insight into the emergence of education for midwives at the turn of the century. She has also been involved in more contemporary issues related to postnatal care as a member of the WHO Technical Working Group and the NICE guideline development group for England and Wales.

Christine McCourt is professor of anthropology and health at Thames Valley University, based in the Centre for Research in Midwifery and Childbirth (CeMaC). Her key interest at doctoral level was in applying anthropological theory and methodology to studying 'western' health-care. Since then, her main work has been on maternity and women's health, with particular interests in institutions and service change and reform, on women's experiences of childbirth and maternity care and in the culture and organisation of maternity care. She published and presented widely in these areas. She is a member of the ICM (International Congress of Midwives) research standing committee and managing editor of the international applied anthropology journal *Anthropology in Action*.

Selina Nylander taught science and health and social care for 5 years before retraining as a public health analyst in 2006. She is currently working as a researcher for Liverpool University and completing a Masters dissertation on physiological birth (Incidence and Outcomes).

She has been a member of Liverpool National Childbirth Trust for 5 years and has been a breast pump agent, fundraiser, chair, MSLC representative and research representative. She has run a homebirth support group in Liverpool for 4 years and has recently become the lead for a research users group at Liverpool Women's Hospital. She has been a recognised birth doula with Doula UK since 2006.

In 2008 she was appointed as a lay supervisory area reviewer for the Nursing and Midwifery Council. She has recently set up a consultancy (http://www.deverra.co.uk) specialising in physiological birth and risk.

Christine Shea works in safety and risk management specifically in the management of safety and risk in complex, safety-critical domains such as health care, aviation, rail and petroleum industry. Her research interests include the management and organisation of work in safety-critical domains, safety culture, the development and implementation of incident reporting systems and human error. She began her career in safety and risk, conducting research in Accident and Emergency departments and neonatal intensive care units specifically investigating the interactions between the organisation of work, technology and human factors and the impact of these on safety and risk. She is now applying these skills and experience to birth. Christine has been involved in her local National Childbirth Trust and homebirth group for the last 4 years. Pulling all of this work together Christine has recently set up a consultancy (www.deverra.co.uk) to conduct research, provide information and raise awareness on risk and physiological birth.

Jane Yelland is a research fellow in the Healthy Mothers Healthy Families research group at the Murdoch Children's Research Institute in Melbourne, Australia. She has a background in nursing and women's health and has spent the last 20 years in research. She has a keen interest in maternal health, cross-cultural research and health services research.

Jane was an investigator on the first Australian study to review hospital-based postnatal care. She is currently an investigator on a population-based survey of recent mothers in South Australia and Victoria; a 'sister' study to the survey, the Aboriginal Families Study and a study piloting a new approach to early postnatal care at a Melbourne hospital.

Chapter 1
The History of Postnatal Care, National and International Perspectives

Sally Marchant

The Princess was composed after her delivery, and, though of course much exhausted, every hope was entertained of her doing well. A little after twelve a change was observed in Her Royal Highness. Her quiet left her – she was restless and uneasy, and the medical attendants felt alarmed. From half-past twelve restlessness and convulsions increased, till nature and life were quite exhausted, and Her Royal Highness expired at half-past two this morning.

(Jones 1885)

Introduction

The history behind the role of midwives and their sphere of practice has already been comprehensively described in a number of publications (Schnorrenberg 1981; Donnison 1988; van Teijlingen 2004). These texts describe how the attendance of the midwife, particularly to a woman in labour, has often been undertaken within a framework of conflict, tension and disharmony by a whole range of key figures in society. These include representatives of the main religions as well as most male medical practitioners. The impact of these influences on the work of midwives was very mixed, with some midwives gaining considerable skills and knowledge from working with doctors (van Teijlingen 2004) while others had less formal training and, where they often used a range of traditional remedies, they were viewed with suspicion and, to some extent, disdain (Donnison 1988; Southern 1998). It was only comparatively recently, considering the longevity of the work of midwives in society, that there was a more objective recognition of their role leading to professional recognition and registration (Cowell & Wainwright 1981; Donnison 1988).

While there is quite extensive literature on the work of the midwife when attending women in labour, there is less detailed information about what was expected of the midwife with regard to the care of the mother and the new baby after the birth had taken place. This lack of information hampers the interested researcher trying to tease out the more specific role of the midwife in relation to post-birth care and overall maternal and infant health. However, based on the contemporary textbooks and other literature available, this chapter will explore the status of the midwife and the role given to post-partum care and how it has evolved over the centuries but mainly within the context of care provision in the United Kingdom at the time the Midwives Act was passed in 1902. The main focus for the text will be on the relationship of the health and well-being of the mother and the care provided to her after birth. This will be addressed in terms of management of care for the most serious aspects of ill health post-partum, rather than in relation to the entire range of possible post-partum health problems. Care of the newborn is not included in this chapter.

Historical references to midwifery and post-birth care

There is evidence that midwifery as a female occupation was recognised in ancient Egypt between the period 1900 and 1550 BC as it is included in some of the text identified from the *Ebers papyrus Encyclopaedia Britannica* (2008). In ancient Egypt, midwifery was a recognised female occupation as verified in another text, the Westcar papyrus, and it would appear that midwifery was a well-recognised aspect in this culture (Chamberlain 1981; Towler & Bramall 1986). Midwives are also evident in Greek and Roman times, although their professional status is not entirely clear (De Costa 2002). Some texts suggest that midwives could be quite well educated, to the extent that they were then seen as medical physicians (French 1986). They used a wide range of herbal and other remedies in their practice and received payment for their work. However, where families could not afford the fees of these more educated midwives they appear to have been attended by other unskilled women who used a more dubious range of practices (Flemming 2000). Some midwives may have originally been slaves but it would appear where they could receive some payment for their work, it is possible that they were then able to buy their freedom, thereby achieving a more respected status in Roman Society (Flemming 2000).

On the demise of the Roman Empire and the emergence of Christianity, the work of midwives came to the attention of the Church (De Costa 2002) There are similarities between several of the main religions with regard to events after childbirth for both the mother and the new infant. In particular, the period of recovery after the birth appears in most cultures and is linked to religious rituals, although the duration of this period varies. A wide range of customs and rituals have been adopted but many appear to be underpinned by concerns over the woman's spiritual integrity and the need for her to undertake some form of cleansing as well as a period of recovery after the birth (Kitzinger 2000; Cartwright Jones 2002).

Focusing on mainland Europe, the Catholic Church appears to have had concerns about the need to have control over a woman's fertility and her influence on men (Biggar 1972; Ehrenreich & English 1973; Derbyshire 1985). It was generally considered that the pains of labour were entirely justified since all women were descendents of Eve and that they should 'pay' the consequences of Eve having led Adam astray. The work of midwives was therefore regarded with some suspicion where they had access to women for a range of conditions linked to sex often in preference to care from physicians or male healers. Where they then used a range of herbal remedies to relieve the pain of labour, this, in effect, was going against the will of God (Southern 1998; van Teijlingen 2004). This was in an era when good and evil were strong paradigms used to explain the causes of disease and death by attributing the outcomes to either salvation by God or damnation by the Devil. In order to exert some control over these 'women's affairs' the Church became involved in deciding who was fit to be a midwife by introducing a form of licensing. This was undertaken by a bishop and the midwife was required to swear an oath not to use magic when assisting women through labour (Field 1993; Wiesner 2004).

The emergence of male midwives and of the involvement of doctors in midwifery, as opposed to obstetrics, is not discussed here as the care of the lying in woman and her infant was almost entirely the province of women, unless complications required the assistance of a medical practitioner, where this could be afforded (Schnorrenberg 1981; Donnison 1988).

Historical aspects of care and support post-birth and its relevance to current health provision

However far back history takes us with regard to care after childbirth, it would appear that the main reason for maternal death then, as it is today in many parts of the world, was infection and haemorrhage and the interrelationship between the two. The post-partum period or puerperium describes the time after the birth where recovery takes place in the major organs and the body systems return to their pre-pregnant state, apart from the hormonal cycle, where the influence of prolactin for breastfeeding affects the production of oestrogen and progesterone, reducing the woman's level of fertility. The time frame for these occurrences has traditionally been around 6 weeks, or 40 days and as such, as noted previously, also appears to have been incorporated into many religious and social frameworks for motherhood and care of the new mother and her child (Southern 1998). The process of birth, especially where the mother continued to have vaginal bleeding or fluid loss, was treated with great suspicion and anxiety. In many religions, the woman was considered unclean until the vaginal loss had ceased. This time frame was linked to the sex of the baby and would have an effect on the length of time the woman was excluded from social and religious events, until such time as she could be 'cleansed' (Southern 1998).

This also meant that in some social settings, men were discouraged or even forbidden from being in contact with their wives and newly delivered babies for several days or weeks after the birth. This in turn also fuelled suspicion around the activities of the women, the new mother, and those who attended her, where there was doubt over the viability of the child as well as the health of the mother (Cartwright Jones 2002).

It is not possible in this chapter to explore these issues in great detail, but it is important to note that many of the customs undertaken today that have their origins from many centuries ago remain significant to the members of those cultures.

Good practice point: reflection exercise: historical aspects of post-partum care and current practice

It may be helpful to consider how well you know the social circumstances of the woman you are attending post-natally. Where some cultures have preferences for foods and rituals, how well does the care you are providing account for these? An example is where there is a naming ceremony for the baby – did you know about this? If not, you might have kept on asking the baby's name before this has been given to him, you might also have arranged a visit on the day of the ceremony.

Where there was perhaps an overemphasis on rest – particularly, that of enforced bed rest, the situation is not very different and arguably, new mothers do not seem to think they need much 'daytime' rest, but then they are deprived of sleep overnight. How do you help a new mother manage her rest periods, how do you explain about rest and time for herself where she is breastfeeding? There are only the two of them and they are anxious about the care of their baby. What resources could you offer them to improve the situation?

Life and death – midwives as helpers of God or the Devil

Infection poses one of the greatest threats to women's health after the birth. References to 'childbed fever' have been found in old Hindu texts and in the writings of Hippocrates and these identify the extreme concern attached to this where there was such a high risk of death (De Costa 2002). There was also some understanding of the basic nature of infection and that this disease could be passed on to other women, although the mechanism and identification of bacteria was not recognised until many centuries later. There appears to be very scant literature regarding the work of midwives attending women at the birth or afterwards throughout the early times of Christianity and into the Middle Ages. This might reflect that many midwives would not have had access to writing materials, or been able to read or write, and even if they did write this down, it is not clear who would have read it. The impression from one of the earliest English texts is that the work of the midwife was one that was passed down and that the midwife was expected to rely on experience and possibly, trial and error (Fraser 1984).

The frequency of maternal death from infection 'childbed fever' and the lack of knowledge about what caused it may have contributed to an overtly polarised religious framework of the work of God versus the work of the Devil. This led to great suspicion of the activities of women and the work of midwifery and threatened the control that could be achieved by the established Church. Midwives fitted both aspects of a spectrum by being called 'wise women' undertaking the work of God by assisting the safe birth of new life, to being 'witches' involved in the work of the Devil (Ehrenreich & English 1973). As witches, midwives were also seen as being responsible for a wide range of social ills related to sex, conception and abortion as can be seen from a text listing the main 'crimes' of witches that underpins the great suspicion about the powers of which many midwives were then accused of:

> Now there are, as it is said in the Papal Bull, seven methods by which they infect with witchcraft the venereal act and the conception of the womb: First, by inclining the minds of men to inordinate passion; second, by obstructing their generative force; third, by removing the members accommodated to that act; fourth, by changing men into beasts by their magic act; fifth, by destroying the generative force in women; sixth, by procuring abortion; seventh, by offering children to the devils, besides other animals and fruits of the earth with which they work much charm . . .
>
> (Malleus Maleficarum in Kramer & Sprenger 1928)

Post-partum treatments and rituals in the Middle Ages

Where midwives used a range of herbs and plant extracts as healing agents, these were called *witches brews* despite their ability, in some cases, to heal rather than harm the women (Biggar 1972; Ehrenreich & English 1979). There was also use of incantations and talismans, all of which raised suspicion during this period of religious fervour where there was a need to find someone on earth to blame for the actions of God or of the Devil and where death was such a frequent visitor to so many households. From the fourteenth to the seventeenth century in the main cities of Europe, this suspicion led to many midwives being branded as witches and being put to death, although this was less common in England (van Teijlingen 2004; Wiesner 2004). Historical writers reflecting on this time suggest that it was incumbent upon the key figures of society, both religious leaders and medical men, to try to make sense of these events although the Church and medicine were at some conflict themselves (Ehrenreich & English 1973). Therefore, to some extent, midwives were the perfect solution to fill that need where they had almost sole access to childbearing women and where, of course, they were women.

Where the midwife was seen as the 'wise woman', she was usually a local woman of more mature years, was usually married and had given birth herself (Wiesner 2004). These women offered their skills in attending women in childbirth and often received no overt payment for this. Prior to the extreme suspicion and witch hunts of midwives, the established Catholic Church had already required midwives to be involved in law enforcement where this concerned conception, pregnancy and childbirth. Midwives were used as 'expert witnesses' for a number of situations, examples including confirming a pregnancy to mitigate the death penalty where a woman had committed a crime as well as to ascertain virginity or impotence in a prospective bride or husband or evidence of a pregnancy where abortion was suspected (Weisner 2004). The Church also involved midwives in post-birth rituals where it was the midwife who presented the infant for baptism at the christening and who was also part of the female group that gossips at the ceremonial churching of the post-partum mother. Churching was a ceremony undertaken to purify the woman's defilement of carrying the unconsecrated fetus and was performed around 6 weeks after the birth when the woman was also considered to be free from the pollution of uterine blood (Donnison 1988; Newell 2007). Baptism of the infant was an essential part of mediaeval Catholicism. If there was insufficient time to get a dying child baptised by a priest, it was considered appropriate that the midwife should do so to ensure that the infant would not be consigned to remain forever in purgatory (Wiesner 2004). The midwife would be instructed not only on the correct words to use, according to the religious laws at the time but also to ensure that no subversive or satanic incantations were used instead. If there was any suspicion of this, the midwife would be removed from practice. Various artefacts from the birth including the placenta, membranes and umbilical cord, were all considered to have mystical (benevolent and malevolent) as well as healing powers and the midwife was involved in either the protection of these or in their appropriate disposal. This again placed the midwife in a position apart from the medical men or church leaders of the time, fuelling the concern for being linked with the work of the Devil.

From some contemporary notebooks, it can be seen that the midwives and physicians used a range of resources to ward against haemorrhage and sickness after the birth. In her detailed account of midwifery during this time, Jane Sharp gives detailed accounts of what action should be taken to assist the haemorrhaging woman (Hobby 1999). While it is of perhaps rather morbid interest to note what was used, these 'remedies' included a range of substances. For example, to reduce the risk of haemorrhage it was advised to use poultices and suppositories of hogs dung and ashes of toad, as well as laying a newly flayed sheep skin over the abdomen to assist in the delivery of the 'after burden' (Hobby 1999). Donnison (1988) in her seminal publication on midwifery history comments that Jane Sharp's adherence to such practices noted above were founded on superstition and poor knowledge, and were no longer in use by other contemporary midwives. However, the list of remedies recounted by Jane Sharp and the observations of physical disorder (uterine prolapse, oedema, infection) demonstrate how much concern and diligence was held about the services a midwife could offer to relieve women's pain and distress associated with pregnancy, childbirth and the puerperium (Hobby 1999). Therefore, in some instances, treatments are noted that are still in common use today – an example being fennel to ease gastric pain in the infant.

Good practice point

There is a wide choice of conventional and alternative medicines available to help women feel more comfortable with their own health and that of their baby after they have given birth. Examples of proprietary products include paracetamol, lactulose, Lansinoh and Co-relief, as well as a huge range of skin lotions and creams, and, of course, formula milk. What framework would you use in deciding what advice you can give a new mother who is considering using these products, with regard to benefits for her health and that of her new baby? What safeguards are in place to reduce the risk of harm from any of these products and why is it important to know about them?

At the same time there were practices that clearly encouraged infection and poor health where, for example, there was great adherence to 'sealing up' the birthing room and where women remained in bed in what could be very overheated rooms for up to 9 days after the birth. Charms or talismans were given to the women in the form of necklets and girdles made of blue thread and worn by the new mother as they were thought to ward away sickness and ensure a good milk supply (Biggar 1972; Hobby 1999). The health of the infant was directly dependent on a healthy mother who could breastfeed; however, where this was not possible, there were alternatives and a range of substances were given to babies who were in need of supplementation (Hobby 1999). Alternatively, there were the services of a wet nurse that was available to some, not always on a payment basis, as women in the community would be likely to offer their services when this was needed (Tait 2003).

Education, enlightenment and the involvement of medical men

Although a more enlightened age evolved after the Middle Ages, the prevalence of childbed fever continued unabated. As a result of the reformation and greater use of written records, albeit usually in Latin, more information could be shared between physicians across Europe and beyond and a more overt scientific community began to be established (Ehrenreich & English 1973; Donnison 1988; van Teijlingen 2004). The first epidemic of puerperal fever was recorded as having occurred in Paris in 1646, where one woman in four died following childbirth. Such high levels of mortality appear to have led to the setting up of 'lying in' hospitals around the seventeenth century where labouring women could be attended by midwives and obstetricians and where the aim was to give greater care for women in labour and for a designated time afterwards (Mackenzie 1872). However, far from improving the care women received in labour, the 'lying in' hospitals were often grossly overcrowded, instruments were reused unwashed, blood-soaked and contaminated linen was also reused and the high frequency of internal examinations led to increased infection rates, making these institutions places more of death than of life. In addition, there was still poor understanding of the physiology of the puerperium and some confusion over what was termed *mental disarray* alongside physical disorders, which hindered appropriate treatment. 'Mental disarray' of course could have presented where very high temperatures from puerperal infection led to disorientation, as well as from the known hormonal factors associated with the immediate post-partum period.

The term *lying in* then seems to have been adopted to describe the time of labour itself and then for a designated time afterwards where women could 'recover' and nurse their newborn. This will be referred to later in the chapter when discussing instructions for the attendance of midwives at the beginning of the twentieth century.

While Semellweiss is usually given the accolade for having been the first to link contamination between care attendants and women as the source of puerperal infection, it appears a Dr Oliver Wendall Holmes had actually proposed this connection a few years earlier in America in 1843 (De Costa 2002). His initial theories were ridiculed by his peers; however, his work and of course, the work of Semmelweiss became a turning point in the recognition of contamination and the onset of disease, although it took almost 40 years before there was general acceptance of this from the scientific and medical fraternities (De Costa 2002).

Other medical discoveries also contributed to better understanding of puerperal sepsis where the need for a clean environment and how to obtain this were identified by Lister in the mid-nineteenth century (Illingsworth 1964) followed by the identification of bacteria by Pasteur in 1879. Therefore, while doctors were now more conversant with the aetiology of infection, they were not, on the whole, the people who had the most contact with childbearing women, most of whom continued to be attended by midwives.

Life-threatening blood loss

Haemorrhage, either immediately after the birth or within the post-natal period, is still one of the main causes of maternal death and contributes to longer term morbidity in the puerperium. Where women approach childbirth in poor physical health, especially where they are anaemic, undernourished or with a pre-existing infection, then even small amounts of blood loss at the birth can seriously affect their health. Where catastrophic haemorrhage occurs, the management for this, to some extent, still remains outside the management or control of carers in the twenty-first century, let alone at the time preceding blood transfusions or the current methods available to maintain circulatory support. There is less information in the literature about treatment for excessive or prolonged blood loss, which is surprising considering the emphasis placed on lochia in the rituals surrounding the puerperium.

In this chapter, I will concentrate on secondary post-partum haemorrhage, which lies more in the remit of postnatal care within the community setting than primary haemorrhage (largely covered in Chapter 6).

The effect on postnatal care of formalising midwifery as a profession

It was around the mid-nineteenth century when the Victorian era of enlightenment was at its peak, that more women began to emerge as campaigners for the status of women in society as a whole. It also needs to be acknowledged that there were many influential men also working for the improvement of social welfare. These included such diverse people as Dr John Snow who identified the cause of cholera from the appalling state of London's sewers (Frerichs 2009) as well as Charles Dickens, whose writings brought the social inequalities into the public eye.

Care of women following childbirth, where there was no formal recognition of the midwife, led to a wide range in those who offered their services to the post-partum woman and her family – from the appearance of the frankly drunken midwife, Sarey Gamp, as portrayed by Dickens (1844) in his book *Martin Chuzzlewit* and supported by other publications of the era (Haslem 1996), to the slightly less malevolent references made to what was called the 'handywomen'. There was also the more official employment of the 'monthly nurse', and of course, there was still the midwife (Leap 1993). Whether these women had midwifery skills or were unskilled women who were willing to take care of a new mother and her baby for payment, is unclear, although from various contemporary texts, it would appear that the monthly nurse (who could be a midwife as well as a nurse or also be untrained) would move into the family home for the 4 weeks after the birth and help with household duties as well as caring for the mother (Donnison 1988; Leap 1993).

This lackadaisical state of affairs was not in keeping with the still high rates of maternal and infant deaths in the first few weeks after childbirth and the emerging recognition of the need for better social welfare. This was a time of great social introspection and as a result of this, small advances were made on behalf of women, where, for example, it was recognised that the work of caring for the sick required some instruction above just kindness or necessity. This led to the instigation of a formal nursing education and with regards to midwifery, the attainment of a diploma from the London Obstetrical Society (Cowell & Wainright 1981). In the United Kingdom, following her own nurse training, Florence Nightingale, while being best known for her work in the Crimea, also had a huge influence on improving public health services (Nightingale 1871; Dunn 1996; Baly 1997). Her work with government officials influenced the organisation of services that aimed to reduce the high levels of poor health caused by poverty and ignorance. She was also supportive of the actions of Zepherine Veitch and others in their campaign to establish some form of regulation and training for midwives (Cowell & Wainwright 1981).

From the perspective of midwifery, Zepherina Veitch was one of the most influential women to promote the education of midwives and her collaboration with Louisa Hubbard, a journalist, led to the setting up of the Trained Midwives Registration Society as the forerunner to the Midwives Institute and ultimately, The Royal College of Midwives

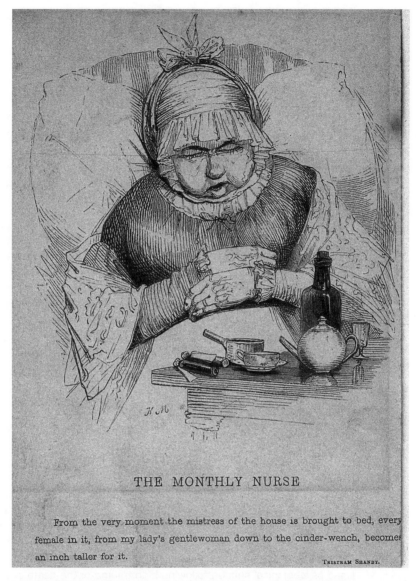

THE MONTHLY NURSE

From the very moment the mistress of the house is brought to bed, every female in it, from my lady's gentlewoman down to the cinder-wench, becomes an inch taller for it.

TRISTRAM SHANDY.

The monthly nurse. Taken from the Wellcome Library, London, by kind permission of the Wellcome Trust.

(Cowell & Wainwright 1981). Such leadership motivated other women who were well placed in society to make a difference (Heagerty 1997). Women with common aims to improve women's status in society met through a range of societies, one such being the Co-operative Guild (Llewellyn Davies 1990). These societies advised and supported women from a range of social backgrounds to cope with a life often of great poverty, but also giving them vision for a better future (see Box 1.1).

Box 1.1 Memoirs of Mrs Layton, bonafide midwife

Mrs Layton recalls her life and how she became a bonafide midwife, from initially being asked to help at several births because the women could not afford a midwife. She considered training to be a midwife but could not afford the £30 needed to fund her training. She was very experienced and as part of her practice, worked alongside several doctors who appeared to recognise her skills, lent her textbooks and even instructed her on the use of forceps. She did eventually attempt to train as a midwife but sadly failed the exam and was instead admitted to the roll as a bonafide midwife when the Midwives Act was passed in 1902 ('Memories of seventy years' by Mrs Layton in Llewellyn Davies (1990), p. 35–55).

The focus on education and the need to regularise the work of midwives became an important goal for many women at that time although the pathway to achieving such registration was long and arduous, and was met with considerable opposition from both medical and nursing contemporaries (Donnison 1988). It is perhaps a throw back from these days that there is still a degree of antagonism rather than collaboration between midwives and obstetricians; where there was such opposition to something that should have meant better standards of care for women overall.

Good practice point

This point relates to the role of all health-care professionals and possibly other health-care workers in what care is available to women after they have given birth. You might want to think through the different aspects of post-partum care; these might include the need for direct care to relieve pain, the need for nursing care to reduce the risk of ill health from infection or complications following surgery, of information needs about child care, and psychological support following birth trauma or the death of a baby. At some point, it is possible that a woman will need care and support from a number of health workers, professional and non-professional. What aspects of direct and indirect care would you consider to be common to everyone involved? What would improve or reduce the effectiveness and satisfaction for the woman?

The eventual passing of the Midwives Act in 1902 in England set the future framework not only for the education and standards to be attained by midwives but also for a recognised framework of care provision for pregnancy, labour and birth, and afterwards (Donnison 1988; van Teijlingen 2004). The setting up of the Central Midwives Board allowed for the provision of regulations that set out the required standards and tasks that were to be undertaken by midwives. In comparison with the broad base of our current rules and standards (NMC 2004), these are highly detailed and specific with regard to what was expected from the certified midwife (Calder 1912; Central Midwives' Board 1919; Berkeley 1924) A number of contemporary textbooks set out the rationale for some of these activities and it would appear that these were, and to some extent still are, led by the concern over the risk of illness and death following childbirth, as opposed to recovery and restoration to normal health (Longridge 1906; Calder 1912; Berkeley 1924).

International aspects of midwifery regulation and registration

Midwives in Europe were also keen to collaborate and there are records of a conference held in Berlin and attended by 1000 midwives from Europe (ICM 2008). The origins of what is now the International Confederation of Midwives are said to have begun in Antwerp in 1919 when midwives from several European countries met on a regular basis. There are very few records for the period before and during the World War II, but in 1954, another meeting was convened in London and this was the point when the name of the International Confederation of Midwives was decided and the framework for the triennial Congresses established (Towler & Bramall 1986).

In the United States, while there had always been 'lay' or untrained midwives (Humphrey 1891) the Frontier Nursing Service, led by Mary Breckenridge introduced a training for nurse-midwives in 1925 (Centre for Nursing Advocacy 2008). This was broadly based on the UK midwifery model of both nursing and midwifery instruction. From these beginnings, a more established national service was promoted and the Frontier Graduate School of Midwifery started the first nurse-midwifery education programme in 1939 to produce 'certified' nurse-midwives (Centre for Nursing Advocacy 2008).

Certified nurse-midwives were educated in both nursing and midwifery to provide gynaecological and midwifery care in recognised institutions as well as in women's homes. There continued to be lay midwives, uncertified or unlicensed midwives who obtained their skills through more informal routes such as self-study or apprenticeship rather than through a formal programme. However, as with the health services in the United Kingdom, the increasing involvement of medicine and doctors in matters associated with normal childbirth alongside the establishment of formal certification of midwives meant that very few untrained midwives continued to practise, and there was increasing inequality in the provision of care to non-white women in America (Bair & Caylett 1993).

This picture of the midwife with skills but no formal qualifications is replicated throughout the world as the recognition of education and formal training, and its beneficial impact on mortality and morbidity was recognised (Field 1993). Where, over recent years, there have been considerable efforts to reclaim the origins and identity for midwifery as a separate and discrete profession from nursing, it is difficult to fully understand the background that meant so much to those campaigners for registration and reformers of the health services, such as they were, over 100 years ago.

Once the regulation and registration of midwives was achieved in any country, this set the pathway for midwifery registration up to the present day. While there have been considerable changes in presentation of the role and scope of practice for midwives, there remains a statutory obligation in the United Kingdom to attend the mother and child for a set period after the birth. The next section will address the content of care expected of midwives from the late nineteenth to early twentieth century. It is by understanding some aspects of this framework for care that the current challenges and dilemmas facing contemporary postnatal care can be assessed (see Chapter 2).

Historical aspects of post-partum care and clinical observations

As noted earlier, puerperal infection and haemorrhage were lethal conditions for the post-partum mother (Loudon 1987) and the role of the midwife was to observe for signs that might indicate the mother was either at increased risk of developing this major morbidity or was already affected. There was a strong adherence to the need for the new mother to rest and to remain in bed, lying down, for a set number of days before they could even sit up, and then stay in bed for a further few days before being allowed to sit in a chair and eventually to walk about. This, of course, was only possible for those who were not required to work or provide for their family's needs, and who could afford the attendance of the midwife and/or the monthly nurse (Donnison 1988). The work of the midwife varied from being a professional attendee to also undertaking basic household chores and activities in order to allow the women to stay in bed. The monthly nurse was seen more as an attendant for the mother and carer of the new infant (see Box 1.2).

Box 1.2 Qualifications of a monthly nurse

1. A good nurse ought not only to be a woman of irreproachable moral character, but she ought to also have a deep sense of religion. This will lead her to regard her office as a high vocation, the duties of which are to be conscientiously performed for His sake, who entrusted them to her; it will support her under fatigue, and in the midst of scenes of difficulty, distress, and sorrow, will lead her to the only source of strength, and comfort and wisdom. An irreligious nurse will generally be more or less inefficient.
2. She ought to possess a tender sympathy for the sufferings of others; far from interfering with her usefulness, this will render her efforts more diligent and untiring, at the same time that the gentleness and feeling she manifests will soothe the patient and acquire her confidence.
3. A habit of quick yet careful observation is essential, lest she should overlook some important symptom, or undervalue some unusual occurrence, and so lose the earliest opportunity of affording relief, or of sending for advice and assistance.
4. She should possess a certain amount of education. A nurse who cannot read cannot be trusted with the administration of medicines without great risk; but a degree of cultivation ensures greater intelligence, and, as they have abundant leisure, they have time for improvement. I can also say, from experience, that a nurse who can read pleasantly has it in her power to beguile many a weary hour for her patient.
5. Neatness and cleanliness should characterise not only her person and dress, but the entire sphere of her duties. The arrangements of the sick chamber, of the bed, of the patient and of the infant, should all be marked by order, cleanliness and neatness. A slatternly nurse is generally something worse. She should have 'a place for everything, and everything in its place'. (Churchill 1872)

From the midwife's viewpoint, the spectre of death from disease and excessive blood loss was ever present, and a number of observations were undertaken on a regular and consistent basis to alert the midwife to the possibility of complications and make referral to a medical practitioner where this was appropriate. The observations included palpation of the uterus to assess the rate of involution and recording maternal temperature and pulse and on occasions, the respiration rate. The state of the breasts and the activities around breastfeeding and bladder and bowel function would also be noted. The woman's psychological well-being was also observed, although it has been argued that the assessment of this was often dubious and critically flawed (Marland 2004). The next part of this chapter explores the advice given to midwives on post-partum care, based on the information presented in textbooks written for midwives early in the last century. The textbooks offer quite detailed descriptions of aspects of post-partum care, including how to perform abdominal palpation of the post-partum uterus and advice that such observations should be carried out at the same time of day and by the same attendee (Longridge 1906; Calder 1912; Berkeley 1924). The authors of the textbooks were medical practitioners who not only made up the majority of members of the newly created Central Midwives Board who issued the instructions that regulated midwifery care, but were also largely responsible for presenting the lectures that led to certification.

Good practice point

'A silly ritual of measuring the height of the fundus of the uterus above the symphysis pubis carried on. It was charted daily as if it gave an indication of the rate of involution. The measurement is only in one dimension, whereas, involution is three-dimensional. It wasted a lot of time to no purpose'. (Rhodes 1995, p. 170–171)

What do you think about the above statement? Do you generally agree or disagree with it? Whatever your decision, give at least two reasons to support your view and how this is reflected in current practice in the United Kingdom.

The examination of the post-partum uterus can offer valuable information about the progress of involution and the return of the uterus as a pelvic organ. However, there is a need to accommodate the information gained from your palpation with a range of other clinical observations in order to make an overall assessment of normality. What would you consider to be the most important information to help you make your decision?

Care of the post-partum woman

Attendance of a midwife

When the first Midwives Act was passed in 1902, a framework was set for the duties and obligations of the midwife, during a woman's pregnancy, labour and puerperium. The 'lying in' period was defined as the period of labour and the 10 days following this and the midwife was responsible for 'the cleanliness and give all necessary directions for securing the comfort and proper dieting of the mother and child'

(Calder 1912). Most births took place in the home, and the midwife would visit within 12 hours of labour, once daily for first 3 days, thereafter every other day until a woman got up. Generally women were very much 'confined; to bed where their social circumstances could support this' (Baker 1985). Instructions about the length of time women should remain in bed are quite specific although a link is made to the physical recovery of the woman where they may mobilise earlier if involution is complete and the lochia have ceased. Generally though the following extract is typical of the advice regarding bedrest:

> Rest in the horizontal position is essential to the lying in if the double results of involution are to be accomplished. The rest should continue at least a month, the first two weeks in bed, then one week out of bed lying on the sofa, and the fourth in the bedroom, lying down at intervals.
>
> (Calder 1912, p. 130)

> The usual practice is to keep the patient in bed during the nine days subsequent to labour. Some authorities advocate fourteen days on the assumption that this additional rest tends to reduce uterine displacements and sub-involution, complications more particularly found in women of the poorer classes.
>
> (Berkeley 1924, p. 380)

It is fascinating to read some of these texts where the authors almost debate with themselves about the wisdom of certain actions. With regard to the involuting uterus and the freedom of drainage of the lochia, one author questions the wisdom of such prolonged periods of bedrest as this would only promote the retention of fluid rather than assist its discharge, but then seems to dissuade himself of this notion, considering it only for women of the 'lower classes'. Having recommended the framework of rest over the first month Calder (1912) then debates these new practices and their safety for women overall as this extract shows:

> Many patients it is true, leave their beds long before this, and apparently without harm, making it difficult to convince them of the risk they run; but bad results must frequently follow as is shown in any outpatient department for women's diseases. Attempts have been made in some quarters to get the civilised woman to do as the uncivilised does, and not to lie up for the usual time, but so far the results have not proved that this is a safe plan to follow.
>
> (Calder 1912, p. 130)

Reading these textbooks written at the cusp of the nineteenth and into the early twentieth century, and on which the early education of future midwives was based, there are also references made to the overall health of the woman according to her social status. Reference is also made to the different social status of the women midwives would attend; therefore women who were in domestic service, or in extreme poverty were recognised as having quite separate health needs from women in situations of greater affluence (Calder 1912; Loudon 1986; Donnison 1988). As can be seen from the following extract, this meant that they would be offered different foods and different advice on the duration of bed rest after childbirth. It is interesting that this advice showed considerable sympathy for the plight of women of lower social class alongside almost a degree of disdain for the pampered, 'well off' woman in her comfortable home.

> In poor circumstances she should be kept in bed for twelve to fourteen days only as this is an opportunity of real rest ... for directly they get up, they have to return to their household duties .... The more comfortably a woman is off, the less time she need spend in bed after her confinement ... she may profitably be allowed to get up a little after the first week.
>
> (Berkeley 1924, p. 381)

In addition to their midwifery duties, midwives were also expected to adhere to the Central Midwives Board guidance, which included a section called *The Principles of Food, Hygiene and Sanitation*. This covered aspects of the woman's social environment where advice from a midwife should include the promotion of health (Calder 1912; Berkeley 1924). A section on sanitation and hygiene is included in both Calder (1912) and Berkeley (1924) although Calder (1912) appears less didactic in giving the following advice:

> It is possible to make a fad of cleanliness without making a fuss of it ... a little tact is required, for it would be unfortunate if the avoidance of dirt meant the avoidance of patients, but with care it is surely possible to keep both cleanliness and a clientele.
>
> (Calder 1912, p. 167)

In Berkeley's (1924) favour is a very relevant instruction that the midwife had an opportunity to work on the woman's behalf where, for example, lodgings were unsuitable and the midwife could notify the local housing authority to improve the living conditions (Berkeley 1924).

As part of the visiting schedule, midwives were clearly expected to be involved in the physical care of the newly delivered woman, by attending to her hygiene needs in the form of a bedbath, of irrigation of the genital area and of seeing to her diet, in some cases, providing and cooking food (Central Midwives' Board 1919; Garcia & Marchant 1996).

Where there existed two 'levels' of midwives in the early part of the twentieth century, it is likely that those who were 'certified' would be more involved with undertaking clinical observations leaving the more direct care and social support in the form of providing food, seeing to some basic household chores and generally offering support to the uncertified midwife or monthly nurse, as described previously (Garcia & Marchant 1996).

Instructions on undertaking specific observations

Uterine involution

Midwives were instructed in the palpation of the uterus to assess the progress of involution; this is clearly described in one extract presented here:

> This is best done by sinking the hand, palm to pubis, into the abdomen above the naval, and bringing it down till it is checked by the fundus.
>
> (Calder 1912, p. 126)

All the text books make reference to the description of a regular descent of the fundus over a period of days post-partum until it is no longer palpable. The text books mostly agree the time period for this as being 10–12 days (Calder 1912; Berkeley 1924). They also offer guidance on when palpation should be undertaken and the action that should be taken when involution was not following the normal pattern. Where recent research has demonstrated such a range of variance with this observation (Cluett *et al.* 1997), it is interesting to note the context within which these observations would have been made at that time. In practice, it probably would be have been the same midwife who would visit at a very similar time each day and this would therefore offer greater consistency with the daily palpations, possibly making them of more value clinically. At one time it was fashionable to bind the uterus, applying a wide strip of cloth around the body and detailed descriptions of how this should be done can be found in the guidance about the role and work of the monthly nurse (Churchill 1872; Berkeley 1924) but this practice was later discarded.

Blood loss

Before blood transfusions were available, the risk of death from haemorrhage was a serious factor in maternal mortality (Loudon 1987). Giving attention to blood loss, with respect to the amount, colour and duration of loss – all feature in the midwifery textbooks alongside information about the midwife's role with regard to cleanliness and disposal of soiled linen. It is advocated that the position of the woman should be lying down in order that 'the lochia drain freely and do not become slightly decomposed, offensive and green' (Calder 1912). Calder's book, *Lectures on Midwifery* (1912), as one of the earliest textbooks gives an account of the make up of the pads used to contain the lochia. These, it is advised, must be 'absolutely aseptic' and this was achieved by putting several of them in a clean bag and placing them in the oven to be 'scorched'. There is also advice on how to make the pads using cheap grey hospital wool encased in cheap muslin, the wool is then discarded and the muslin washed and re-used, with the note that 40 pads could be made for a shilling (Calder 1912). The duration of lochia is noted as being variable, and only tenous links are made to the amount of lochia, colour and the relationship of this to post-partum haemorrhage where there is the presence of blood clots several or few days after the birth. The most significant factor noted in most of the textbooks is a cessation of lochia in the first few days post-partum as a portent of impending uterine infection. Post-partum haemorrhage (both primary and secondary) was treated with what are described as hot douches said to 'stimulate the uterus to contract'. These were of temperatures of at least 115°F up to 120°F and Calder gives the following advice:

> The patient may complain of the heat but if you are certain, by use of a thermometer, it is not greater than 120°F you are not to desist; for a douche cooler than 115°F is lukewarm and of little service, and under 120°F it will not scald. If you do not have a thermometer, water so hot that you cannot keep your hands in it will answer.
>
> (Calder 1912, p. 204)

As well as using the hot douche, it was recommended to knead the uterus to induce a contraction; this was also recommended where there was a possibility of retained products of conception leading to a secondary post-partum haemorrhage (Berkeley 1924). Such measures in contemporary times seem extreme but presumably, where there was little recourse to any other treatment, it was better than watching the woman bleed to death. Although ergot was in use at this time, the midwife was instructed to take all other measures before administering this as it needed time to be effective and was only for use by a midwife in emergency situations. At the time Calder was writing in 1912, the use of saline – a 'teaspoon of common salt in a pint of boiling water' had just been introduced as a method of restoring fluid volume. This was either administered intravenously or rectally by a medical practitioner.

Observations of temperature and pulse

There are quite specific instructions about observing maternal temperature and pulse rate and the relationship of these observations to the development of infection. Calder (1912) notes that the temperature and pulse rate should be taken in the first visit to the post-partum mother in order to establish a baseline for future observations. He also notes that while the pulse rate has been stated to be between 60–70 beats per minute, he suggests it is slightly raised to 75–80 in the days immediately after the birth. The temperature and pulse rate were to be observed night and morning and recorded on a chart. While a small increase in the normal range was acceptable, where this exceeded a degree in Fahrenheit in temperature or a pulse over 90 bpm, then the observations should be repeated in 6 hours, and then repeated over the same time interval until the midwife was certain the temperature was stable and not rising. Where the temperature or pulse rate continued to rise, it was stated that medical assistance must be sought as required by the Central Midwives Rules. Calder (1912) summarises the circumstances where the midwife should seek medical aid:

- Rigour
- Rise of temperature above 100.4°F in 24 hours
- Offensive lochia
- Raised swelling or tenderness in the abdomen, breasts or legs
- Bleeding
- Fits
- Dying or dead

(Calder 1912, p. 248)

All the textbooks included such information although there is also the appreciation that there might be an alternative cause for an increase in temperature other than the development of infection.

The midwife must however, be very careful not to ascribe to some trifling and temporary condition any rise in temperature, since a persistent rise, even though very slight, is nearly always an indication that the patient is septic.

(Berkeley 1924, p. 373)

However, most advice underpins the need for alertness to the presence of infection being the likely cause and that midwives should therefore adhere to the most serious possibility and not dismiss it without due consideration.

Other aspects of care

The textbooks all give quite detailed advice about care of the bladder and bowels, on assistance with breastfeeding as well as management of engorgement, poor lactation and mastitis. There was also great concern about the development of thrombosis, which included the condition called *blue leg* (a venous thrombosis) and *white leg*, which was an infection of the lymphatics (Berkeley 1924). Both conditions could be fatal or lead to long-term morbidity. The instructions for the management of these included minimal movement and prolonged periods of bed rest, demonstrating the lack of understanding of the role of mobilisation and health in circulatory disorders. There is no mention of observation of blood pressure in the early textbooks, and even into the 1950s very little attention was given to taking a blood pressure after the birth although the condition of eclampsia was not uncommon (Gibberd 1943).

Conclusion

This can only be a very limited snapshot into background of key practices and care provision for women following the birth of their baby. While there has been criticism of the content of postnatal care applied on a routine basis with a one size fits all approach (Marchant 2006), it can be appreciated how such patterns of care evolved in an attempt to make childbirth safe for all women, not just the fortunate few. It could be argued that the current status given to the provision of post-birth care, particularly in the developed world, fails to reflect on the huge levels of mortality that was once experienced by many women following childbirth as well as the still quite high levels of morbidity currently reported (Glazener *et al.* 1995; Redshaw *et al.* 2007; Declercq *et al.* 2007). There remains inequality between care provision in countries that have adequate resources compared to those where appropriate resources are not available, resulting in rates of maternal mortality after childbirth that continue to be tragically high. At the same time, contemporary reports suggest that in many developed countries, aspects of postnatal care, in terms of observations of physical recovery as well as psychological and social support, fall short of women's expectations and requirements (Declercq *et al.* 2007; Redshaw *et al.* 2007). The need to understand the complex medical and social issues around early motherhood is essential for the provision of appropriate postnatal care. Therefore, it is no longer the awareness of what causes maternal deaths that is the issue but it is having access to resources that can prevent these events from occurring in the first place that is of most importance. This then gives credibility to reviewing the history of care for women after childbirth where perhaps some of the steps that have been taken to improve women's health can be made more available in locations where resources are scarce, and in other locations where greater recognition of what level and skills from human resources are needed to provide better care for all women and their babies.

Key implications for practice

- There remains considerable disparity in the provision of skilled midwifery care on an international level. Where some countries have a regulated professional framework, others are still struggling for this recognition and this is reflected in the numbers of women who die in childbirth or shortly afterwards. It is therefore important that all midwives acknowledge the work of international groups that are assisting in recognition of midwifery on a worldwide basis.

- Registration as a midwife does not always mean that the care offered is of the highest standard. Midwives in countries where midwifery is a recognised profession cannot afford to be complacent about the care made available to women after they have given birth as not only are there still avoidable instances of morbidity and mortality but there is also increasing feedback from women that what constitutes postnatal care fails to meet their needs with regard to their own health as well as their role as a new mother. As with all aspects of midwifery care, treating women as individuals within a balanced partnership should achieve better outcomes for everyone.

- While the history of the profession might be viewed with a degree of amused tolerance where it is considered care was given without real understanding and clinical knowledge, such an attitude should perhaps be adopted with caution. Women who worked as midwives without the resources we now take for granted made use of those things possibly of most importance in the identification of well-being as well as of potential ill health – their eyes, their hands, their ears and their noses. While the centuries have rolled on, competent midwives should still consider the importance of these, alongside the technology that is available, in reducing maternal ill health after childbirth.

References

Bair B, Caylett S (1993) *Women of Colour and their Experience of Health and Illness in Wings of Gauze*. Detroit: Wayne State University Publication, 202–208.

Baker M (1985) Giving birth in 1872. *Nursing Mirror* 161 (8): 34.

Baly M (1997) *As Miss Nightingale Said*, 2nd Edition. London: Bailliere Tindall, 46, 72, 79–80.

Berkeley C (1924) *A Handbook of Midwifery: for Midwives, Maternity Nurses and Obstetric Dressers*, 6th Edition, Part IV. London: The Puerperium Cassell and Company, Ltd, 370–383.

Biggar J (1972) When midwives were witches . . . white ones of course. *Nursing Mirror*, 36–39.

Calder AB (1912) *Lectures on Midwifery*, 2nd Edition. London: Bailliere Tindall, 121–131, 174–177.

Cartwright Jones C (2002) *Traditional Postpartum Rituals of India, North Africa and the Middle East Kent State University*. www.lotusfertility.com (accessed 18/08/2008).

Central Midwives' Board (1919) *Handbook Incorporating the Rules of the Central Midwives Board*, 5th Edition. London: Central Midwives Board.

Centre for Nursing Advocacy (2008) *The Life of Mary Breckenridge (1881–1965)*. www.nursingadvocacy.org (accessed 16/8/2008).

Chamberlain M (1981) *Old Wives' Tales: Their History, Remedies and Spells*. London: Virago Press.

Churchill F (1872) *Manual for Midwives and Nurses*. Dublin: Fannin and Company.

Cluett ER, Alexander J, Pickering RM (1997) What is the normal pattern of uterine involution? An investigation of postpartum involution measured by the distance between the symphysis pubis and the uterine fundus using a tape measure. *Midwifery* 13: 9–16.

Cowell B, Wainwright D (1981) *Behind the Blue Door: The History of the Royal College of Midwives*. London: Bailliere Tindall.

Declercq ER, Sakala C, Corry MP, *et al.* (2007) Listening to mothers II: report of the second national U.S. survey of women's childbearing experiences. *Journal of Perinatal Education* 16 (4): 9–14.

De Costa CM (2002) The contagiousness of childbed fever: a short history of puerperal sepsis and its treatment. *The Medical Journal of Australia* 177 (11/12): 668–671.

Derbyshire P (1985) Bedpans and broomsticks. *Nursing Times* 81: 44–45.

Dickens C (1844) *Martin Chuzzlewit*. London: Feminist Press.

Donnison J (1988) Chapter 1: The office of midwife: a female mystery 11–33 and Chapter 8: The Midwife's Act. *Midwives and Medical Men*. London: Historical Publications, Ltd, 161–174.

Dunn P (1996) Florence Nightingale (1820–1910): maternal mortality and the training of midwives (Perinatal lesson from the past). *Archives of Disease in Childhood Fetal & Neonatal Edition* 74 (3): 219F–220F.

Ehrenreich B, English D (1973) *Witches, Midwives and Nurses: A History of Women Healers*. London: Feminist Press.

Ehrenreich B, English D (1979) *For Her Own Good: 150 Years of the Expert's Advice to Women*. London: Pluto Press.

Encyclopaedia Britannica (2008) *Ebers Papyruc Encyclopaedia Britannica*. www.britannica.com.

Field P (1993) The context for and nature of midwives in the seventeenth and twentieth centuries. Proceedings of the International Confederation of Midwives 23rd International Congress, Vancouver, Vol. II, 657–661.

Flemming R (2000) *Medicine and the Making of Roman Women*. Oxford: Oxford University Press, 359.

Fraser A (1984) Chapter 22: The modest midwife weidenfield and nicolson. *The Weaker Vessel: Women's Lot in Seventeenth-Century England*. London: Weidenfield and Nicolson.

French V (1986) Midwives and maternity care in the Roman world. *Helios, New Series* 12 (2): 69–84.

Frerichs R on Snow (1813–1858) *UCLA Department of Epidemiology School of Public Health*. http://www.ph.ucla.edu/epi/snow.html (accessed 06/29/2009).

Garcia J, Marchant S (1996) The potential of postnatal care. In: Kroll D (ed). *Midwifery Care for the Future–Meeting the Challenge*, 58–62.

Gibberd GF (1943) Chapter 15: Diseases associated with pregnancy. *A Short Textbook of Midwifery*, 3rd Edition. London: Churchill, 229–230.

Glazener C, Abdalla M, Stroud P, Naji S, Templeton A, Russell I (1995) Postnatal maternal morbidity: extent, causes, prevention and treatment. *British Journal of Obstetrics and Gynaecology* 102 (4): 282–287.

Haslem F (1996) Death in the nursery. *British Medical Journal* 313: 1605.

Heagerty BV (1997) Willing handmaidens of science? The struggle over the new midwife in early twentieth-century England. In: Kirkham MJ, Perkins ER (eds). *Reflections on Midwifery*. London: Bailliere Tindall, 70–95.

Hobby E (ed) (1999) *The Midwives Book or the Whole Art of Midewifery Jane Sharp Oroginally Written 1671*. Oxford: Oxford University Press.

Humphrey M (1891) *The Monthly Nurse: Her Origin, Rise and Progress*. A paper read before the British Nursing Association and published in *The Nursing Record* May 21 1891. www.rcnarchive.rcn.org.uk (accessed 18/08/2008), 267.

Illingsworth C (1964) The Lister Lecture 1964: Wound Sepsis – from carbolic acid to hyperbaric oxygen. *The Canadian Medical Association Journal* 91 (20): 1041–1045.

International Confederation of Midwives (2008) *A Short History of the ICM*. www.internationalmidwives.org (accessed 18/08/2008).

Jones CR (1885) *The Princess Charlotte of Wales, an Illustrated Monograph*, London.

Kitzinger S (2000) *Rediscovering Birth 2000 Sanctuary and Renewal*. London: Little, Brown and Company, 224–238.

Kramer H, Sprenger J (1928) *The Malleus Maleficarum*, translated by Rev. Montague Summers. London: The Pushkin Press.

Leap BH (1993) *The Midwife's Tale: An Oral History from Handywoman to Professional Midwife*. London: Scarlet Press, 1–33.

Llewellyn Davies M (1990) *Life as We Have Known it by Co-operative Working Women*. London: Virago, 38–55.

Longridge CN (1906) *The Puerperium or Management of the Lying-in Woman and Newborn Infant*. London: Adlard and Sons, 95–111, Chapter 5.

Loudon I (1986) Obstetric care, social class, and maternal mortality. *British Medical Journal* 293: 606–608.

Loudon I (1987) Puerperal fever, the streptococcus, and the sulphonamides, 1911–1945. *British Medical Journal* 295: 485–490.

Mackenzie E (1872) *Medical Establishments: The Lying-in Hospital and Charities. Historical Account of Newcastle Including the Borough of Gateshead.* www.british-history (accessed 21/05/2008), 517–522.

Marchant S (2006) The postnatal care journey – are we nearly there yet? *MIDIRS Midwifery Digest* 16 (3): 295–304.

Marland H (2004) Chapter 2: Dangerous motherhood insanity and childbirth in Victorian Britain. *Boundaries of Expertise and the Location of Puerperal Insanity.* Hampshire: Palgrave Macmillan, 35–48.

Newell RC (2007) The thanksgiving of women after childbirth: a blessing in disguise? In: Kirkham M (ed). *Exploring the Dirty Side of Women's Health.* Abingdon: Routledge, 45–59.

Nightingale F (1871) *Notes on Lying in Institutions.* London: Longmans, Green & Company.

Nursing and Midwifery Council (2004) *Midwives Rules and Standards*, Nursing and Midwifery Council 23, Portland, London.

Redshaw M, Rowe R, Hockley C, *et al.* (2007) *Recorded Delivery: A National Survey of Women's Experience of Maternity Care 2006.* Oxford: National Perinatal Epidemiology Unit.

Rhodes P 1995 *A Short History of Clinical Midwifery.* Cheshire, England: Books for Midwives Press. Haigh and Hochland, P 170–P 171.

Schnorrenberg BB (1981) Is childbirth any place for a woman? The decline of midwifery in eighteenth century England. *Studies in Eighteenth Century Culture* 10: 393–408.

Southern J (1998) On trial: women healers. *Midwifery Today Spring*, 35–39.

Tait C (2003) Safely delivered: childbirth, wet-nursing, gossip-feasts and churching in Ireland c. 1530–1690. *Irish Economic and Social History* 30: 1–23, ISSN 03324893.

van Teijlingen ER (2004) History of midwifery: introduction. In: van Teijlingen ER, Lewis GW, McCaffery PG, *et al.* (eds). *Midwifery and the Medicalization of Childbirth: Comparative Perspectives.* Huntington: Nova Science Publishers, 43–51.

Towler J, Bramall J (1986) *Midwives in History and Society.* London: Croom Helm.

Wiesner M (2004) Early modern midwifery: a case study. In: van Teijlingen ER, Lewis GW, McCaffery PG, *et al.* (eds). *Midwifery and the Medicalization of Childbirth: Comparative Perspectives.* Huntington: Nova Science Publishers, 63–74.

Additional Resources

Frerichs on John Snow (1813–1858) BBC. www.bbc.co.uk/history/historic_figures/snow_john.shtml (accessed 20/08/2008).

Ignaz Semmelweis (1818–1865) www.wikipaedia.org (accessed 12/08/2008).

Drainage and Sewage. www.bricksandbrass.co.uk (accessed 8/08/2008).

Chapter 2
Contemporary Postnatal Care in the Twenty-first Century

Debra Bick

Introduction

During recent years the view seems to have been adopted that postnatal care, whilst a core component of midwife practice in the United Kingdom for over a century, is now more of a formality than a public health priority. A number of reasons for this can be postulated. Over the last three decades the long-term trend towards shorter inpatient stay has continued; for example, only 32% of women in 1975 were discharged home within 3 days of giving birth (Richardson & Mmata 2007) while in 2005–2006, 87% of women were discharged within 3 days despite the increase in medical interventions (Richardson & Mmata 2007) and more complex health needs of women who become pregnant (Mander & Smith 2008). Over the same period, domiciliary postnatal contacts have also declined. In 1988–1989, the average rate per maternity in England and Wales was 9.2 postnatal contacts, declining to 7.2 in 1999–2000 (DoH 2000). In a recent survey of women's experiences of maternity care in England in 2006, women received an average of five home visits (Redshaw *et al.* 2007). Despite the need for midwives to optimise the limited number of postnatal contacts they now have with women, there has been a dearth of evidence to support practice. Furthermore, documentation of postnatal care has received limited attention with the implications of how this perpetuates the content of care not being considered, although recent studies of the care pathways to standardise decision-making in labour have commenced this dialogue (Hunter 2007; Rycroft-Malone *et al.* 2008).

The historical, social, cultural and economic influences on women and birth practices since the Middle Ages were described in Chapter 1.

The implications of the introduction in the early twentieth century of midwifery registration and standards for supervision and training were also outlined. One of the most significant catalysts for midwifery and birth practices in the United Kingdom towards the end of the twentieth century was the move for all women to give birth in hospital on the assumption that this was the safest option (Tew 1998). The subsequent impact of the transfer of birth into the acute hospital has impacted on postnatal services because of the need to maximise finite resources, reduce inpatient turnaround intervals and ensure that adequate staffing levels are available on labour wards. As we move into the twenty-first century, we face new challenges of achieving safe, high-quality maternity care following a significant shift in public health priorities, for example, chronic health problems caused by an increasingly obese population in developed countries. While postnatal care has been the subject of recent policy and guideline initiatives, major barriers remain to achieving and sustaining change. In this chapter, the role of postnatal care and its place in meeting twenty-first century public health is addressed, reflecting on evidence, issues and implications for women who give birth in the United Kingdom and internationally.

Developments informing contemporary postnatal care

Despite the introduction of postnatal midwifery care at the beginning of the last century, it was not until the early 1990s that a small number of researchers began to question if the content and timing of routine care were appropriate and policy makers to review how services were organised. The dramatic decline in maternal mortality rates around the time of World War II, followed by the gradual move for all women to give birth in hospital, did not trigger a review of the content or timing of postnatal care. The House of Commons Select Committee Report on the Maternity Services published in 1992 was prompted by widespread concerns about the fragmentation of the maternity services. With respect to postnatal care, the Committee described it as an area that was:

> poorly evaluated and researched, delivered in often inappropriate and fragmented ways and has a dissipated managerial focus which mitigates against effective use of resources. (p. iv)

An Expert Maternity Committee, established in response to the Select Committee Report to examine policy and make recommendations for change, published *Changing Childbirth* (DoH 1993), which was formally adopted as government policy. *Changing Childbirth* (DoH 1993) recommended that research in postnatal care should be broadened, and in redesigning postnatal services, the need for continuity of care should be at the centre. In 1997, The Audit Commission, the official body charged with ensuring how public money is spent, published their report of an external review of the maternity services, which collected data from maternity units, general practitioners (GP) and a survey of women who had given birth in 1995 (Audit Commission 1997; Garcia *et al.* 1998). The report noted the impact that the mother's health on her recovery and adjustment to parenthood and the need to ensure postnatal care was properly planned (Audit Commission 1997).

At the time of publication of these two important reports, little research had been conducted on the content or duration of midwifery postnatal care, which continued to be informed by minimal guidance. Guidance on the duration of contacts included in the 'midwives rules' (UKCC 1998) continued to refer to a period of 'not less than 10 and not more than 28 days after the end of labour during which the continued attendance of a midwife on a mother is requisite', with no evidence to support why this was considered an appropriate length of time to oversee maternal recovery from birth. The content of postnatal care, introduced at the beginning of the twentieth century when prevention of death from haemorrhage and sepsis were a priority, continued to focus on observation of uterine involution, lochia, temperature and blood pressure. This was despite medical advances (e.g. safer anaesthesia, access to contraception and antibiotics to treat puerperal infection), increased awareness of the importance of public health (e.g. better sanitation and housing) as well as advances in the social and economic status of women. A survey of midwifery practice in two English health districts, which examined the content of midwifery home visits, found that although midwives performed traditional components of care on a daily basis, they saw little value in performing them (Garcia *et al.* 1994). An earlier small study of midwifery contacts (Murphy-Black 1989) found that midwives undertook a wide variety of tasks during a home visit but these were frequently not matched to women's needs.

Another traditional component of postnatal care is the routine check with the woman's GP at 6–8 weeks, which marks the end of maternity care. This component of care was introduced around 60 years ago, when the National Health Service was launched, although evidence to support the timing and content of the check is lacking. Despite this being such a routine milestone of a woman's 'journey' through pregnancy and birth, few studies have assessed the benefit of the consultation. Sharif *et al.* (1993) in a small study of 125 women who had routine vaginal examinations at their check found only six had any abnormality detected as a consequence, none of which required treatment. Discussion of contraception at the visit may be too late as women resume sexual intercourse earlier than previously considered

(Glazener *et al*. 1997; Barrett *et al*. 2000). This aspect of postnatal care will be discussed further in the chapter.

Maternal physical and psychological morbidity

One reason for the lack of revision to the timing and content of routine postnatal care was the assumption that performing traditional observations and examinations would detect health problems, and women were physically and psychologically recovered from the birth at the conclusion of postnatal care. The first observational studies of maternal health published in the United Kingdom and Australia (MacArthur *et al*. 1991; Glazener *et al*. 1995; Brown & Lumley 1998) showed that a wide range of maternal physical and psychological health problems were experienced, many of which persisted beyond the postnatal period. Furthermore, health problems were unlikely to be identified within routine postnatal care, as women did not report them and health professionals did not ask about them.

MacArthur *et al*. (1991) in a large study of women who gave birth in one maternity unit in Birmingham, United Kingdom, found that 47% of over 11 000 women reported one or more new health problems occurring for the first time within 6 weeks of giving birth and that many symptoms persisted. A study undertaken in the Grampian region of Scotland found 76% of 1249 women who completed a survey experienced at least one health problem sometime between leaving hospital and the eighth postnatal week (Glazener *et al*. 1997). Commonly reported problems included backache, headaches, fatigue, urinary stress incontinence, haemorrhoids, perineal pain and depression. Studies from Australia, France and Italy reported similar levels of morbidity (Brown & Lumley 1998; Saurel-Cubizolles *et al*. 2000). Furthermore, the impact and severity of health problems was also described for the first time. Whilst problems were not life threatening, some impacted on women's lifestyles and relationships with their family (Bick & MacArthur 1995a,b).

Research has continued to highlight the range and impact of maternal morbidity. Some problems are clearly related to a particular event or intervention during labour or at the time of birth, for example, having a forceps delivery for a first vaginal birth and risk of developing persistent faecal incontinence (MacArthur *et al*. 2005), or having a spinal epidural for labour pain relief and experiencing a post-dural puncture headache (Thew & Paech 2007). Other problems may be related to particular maternal characteristics or the level of social support a woman may have access to; for example, a woman may experience backache because she has no one to assist with caring for her other small children or with lifting heavy shopping or baby equipment (MacArthur *et al*. 1991) or she may have a higher risk of developing depression, based on a previous history of mental health problems or poor marital relationship (NICE 2007).

Although more is known about maternal morbidity now compared with 20 years ago, further primary and secondary research is required to assess the impact on immediate and longer term health issues of pregnancy and birth, including the role of social, cultural and economic factors, and how models of care can be revised to meet needs. It is also important to review clinical training and ongoing staff development to optimise skills to effectively identify and manage postnatal physical and psychological morbidity. Ensuring evidence of benefit is transferred and sustained in practice continues to be a challenge.

Could postnatal care be revised to enhance maternal health?

Following the publication of studies of maternal morbidity, questions were raised about whether routine universal provision of postnatal care could enhance maternal health outcomes and what revisions to care would be necessary to achieve this (MacArthur 1999). Randomised controlled trials (RCTs) undertaken in the United Kingdom and Australia assessed the impact on maternal physical and psychological health of revisions to routine care or an intervention in addition to routine care (see Table 2.1); however, only the RCT by MacArthur *et al.* (2002, 2003) had a positive benefit as described later. RCTs of antenatal or postnatal interventions for women at risk of specific postnatal health problems (i.e. prevention of post-traumatic stress disorder) are not included here.

Midwifery-led postnatal care

The intervention assessed in the RCT by MacArthur *et al.* (2002, 2003) was a package of care delivered by midwives. The unit of randomisation was the general practice. The trial took place across the West Midlands of England and included general practices from rural, urban and inner city areas. The focus of the new model was provision of planned visits over an extended period of time, tailored to women's individual needs with a focus on the identification and management of common health problems. Each woman received a first home visit, a visit at around 10 days and 28 days and a final visit at 10–12 weeks, which replaced the routine GP 6–8 week check. All other visits were to be based on need and not routine, informed by a care plan. Symptom checklists were to be used to identify problems, with evidence-based guidelines for midwives to implement first-line management of those

Table 2.1 Randomised controlled trials of revisions to usual care to enhance maternal postnatal health.

Authors	Intervention	Outcomes	Findings
Turnbull *et al.* (1996) (UK), Shields *et al.* (1997)	Midwife managed antenatal and intrapartum care (*n* = 648) compared with usual care (*n* = 651). Named midwife to lead care. No additions to routine postnatal care	Obstetric intervention (P) Maternal health at 7 weeks (S): EPDS; views of care; satisfaction with care	Fewer antenatal complications (hypertension, haemorrhage), fewer episiotomies, No differences in perineal tears. Birth complications similar, no differences in foetal or neonatal outcomes, EPDS score lower among intervention group
Gunn *et al.* (1998) (Australia)	683 women randomised to early (1 week) postnatal GP visit or usual (6 week) visit, No change to content of visit	EPDS, SF36 at 3 and 6 months (P), breastfeeding, number of problems, satisfaction with GP care (S)	No differences in outcomes. Women randomised to early visit were less likely to attend, more likely to report breastfeeding problems, problems with adjustment to motherhood and less likely to have vaginal examination
Morrell *et al.* (2000) (UK)	Costs and benefits of postnatal support workers. Up to 10, 3-hour visits by support worker in first 28 days (*n* = 311) compared with usual care (*n* = 312)	General health perception domain of SF36 (P). EPDS, Dukes Functional Support Score, breastfeeding (S) at 6 weeks and 6 months	No difference in any health outcomes. Women's satisfaction with support workers higher than for all other services. No savings to NHS
Reid *et al.* (2002) (UK)	2 × 2 factorial trial, community setting. 1004 women randomised – 1. Local support group with facilitator starting 2 weeks post-birth 2. Postnatal handbook posted at 2 weeks post-birth	EPDS score at 3 and 6 months (P) SF36, SSQ6, women's views of care at 2 weeks, 3 and 6 months (S)	Low uptake of support group. No differences in EPDS, SF36 or SSQ6. Women had favourable opinions of the postnatal handbook

Table 2.1 (*continued*)

Authors	Intervention	Outcomes	Findings
MacArthur *et al.* (2002, 2003) (UK)	Cluster RCT of new model of midwifery-led care (*n* = 1087 from 17 GP practices) compared with current care (*n* = 977 from 19 GP practices) Planned midwife visits, symptom checklists at 10 and 28 days, guidelines for management, midwifery care extended to include final check at 10–12 weeks	EPDS scores, mental health domain (MCS) and physical health domain (PCS) of SF36 at 4 and 12 months (P) Breastfeeding, maternal morbidity at 12 months, women's opinions of care, health professionals views of care (S)	Significant difference in EPDS and MCS scores at 4 and 12 months. No difference in physical outcomes. Women's views of care more positive or did not differ. Intervention care was cost-effective

(P) = primary outcome and (S) = secondary outcome

identified. A total of 1087 women were recruited from 17 general practices randomised to the intervention and 977 from 19 general practices, which formed the control group.

Main trial outcomes were the Edinburgh Postnatal Depression Scale (Cox *et al.* 1987), with a score of ≥13 or higher taken as an indication that a woman was likely to be depressed, and the Mental Health Component Score (MCS) and Physical Health Component Score (PCS) of the SF36, a measure of general health and well-being. The outcome measures were included in a postal questionnaire sent at 4 and 12 months after the birth.

Questions on maternal health problems were included in the 12-month questionnaire. Breastfeeding duration was assessed at both time points and 'good' practice indicators such as uptake of infant immunisation were assessed using GP records at 12 months after the birth. A range of process outcome data was also collected to enable the study team to assess if implementation of the new model took place (and which elements were more or less likely to be implemented) and to compare the number of midwifery visits made in the two trial groups for the cost-effectiveness analysis. Women were also asked to keep a diary to record which health professionals had visited them during the postnatal period.

The results showed a significant difference in maternal mental health outcomes at 4 and 12 months after the birth (MacArthur *et al.* 2002, 2003). The distribution of the mean MCS scores by cluster (general practice) showed that the results were general and could not be attributed to one or two clusters with more extreme scores. This was also the case for EPDS scores. There were no differences in PCS scores at either time point. The secondary outcomes that included women's views of care were either significantly more positive in the new model or did not differ between the trial groups. Maternal health problems at 12 months, which were also a secondary outcome, showed significant differences in depression, haemorrhoids and fatigue, which were less likely to be reported by women who received the new model of care, with no difference in breastfeeding outcomes. Women who received the new model of care were less likely to visit their GP during the first year after the index birth about a subsequent pregnancy, and immunisation uptake for the study group showed a 98% uptake. The care provided within the new model was cost-effective as health outcomes were better and costs did not differ substantially.

To date, this is the only trial to have shown a significant effect on maternal postnatal health but only on psychological and not physical health outcomes. Reasons for this could include the difficulty of completely resolving a physical symptom, such as backache or urinary stress incontinence. However, the positive impact on mental health that acknowledgement of a physical symptom could have is also an important consideration. It is also plausible that women who had planned care from a midwife they knew over a longer period of time enabled them to more freely discuss their health.

The trial findings demonstrated for the first time the impact midwives could make to public health from revisions to routine care. The researchers concluded that adaptation of the new model into National Health Service (NHS) care as standard was justified; however, no further work has been undertaken to evaluate if the new model could be implemented outside of a RCT and achieve the same health benefits. Elements of the 'package' of care have been reflected in recent policy such as the National Service Framework for Children, Young People and Maternity Services (DoH 2004) and National Institute for Health and Clinical Excellence (NICE) guidance on routine postnatal care (NICE 2006) but whether this 'piecemeal' approach to postnatal care revision can achieve the same anticipated psychological health benefits is as yet unknown. The next section of this chapter considers recent policy and practice developments for contemporary midwifery postnatal care.

Implications of policy and practice developments on contemporary postnatal care

As referred to earlier, *Changing Childbirth* (DoH 1993) was published following a review of evidence presented to the House of Commons

Select Committee (1992) in response to concerns about the maternity services. There was widespread publicity when the report was published, with many local maternity service providers establishing models of care to meet government targets based on report recommendations, such as ensuring that within 5 years at least 75% of women would know the midwife who cared for them during labour. However, the extent to which implementation of the recommendations was successful is debatable. Where reasons for lack of sustainability were offered, these frequently related to resource and funding issues. Research into pilot projects such as midwifery group practices showed that midwife 'burn-out' was often an issue due to having to provide continuity of care over a 24-hour period to too many women and the role of the multi-professional team in the new models of care was often unclear (Allen *et al.* 1998).

The election of a Labour government in 1997 triggered a major reform of the NHS with the drive to transform it into a service 'fit for the twenty-first century', an end to postcode prescribing, a focus on reducing health inequalities and measures to improve the quality of care, with a particular emphasis on priority areas such as cancer and mental health. Several major policy initiatives were published: some outlining steps to be taken to transform NHS services (DoH 2000), others specifically aimed at reducing poor health (Saving Lives: Our Healthier Nation, DoH 1999), and some targeting specific services including maternity (National Service Framework for Children, Young People and Maternity Services, DoH 2004). A programme of structural and process reform of the NHS was undertaken (Maynard & Street 2006), including the reorganisation of purchasing bodies, the creation of regulatory bodies such as the National Institute for Health and Clinical Excellence and the Care Quality Commission. There have been some key indicators of success, for example, a reduction in waiting times of more than 6 months for elective surgery (Maynard & Street 2006) and evidence that National Service Frameworks have improved the quality of services (King's Fund 2005).

National Service Framework for Children, Young People and Maternity Services

The National Service Framework for Children, Young People and Maternity Services (DoH 2004) was one of the most ambitious and far-reaching policy reports yet published for the maternity services. It included 11 standards for health services relevant to a child's development through infancy, childhood and young adulthood. Standard 11 addresses the requirements of women and their families during pregnancy, birth and the postnatal period, with links to pre- and post-conception health promotion and the Child Health Promotion Programme. The overall standard for maternity care is that:

> Women have easy access to high quality maternity services, designed around their individual needs and those of their babies.

The NSF (DoH 2004) is clear about the importance and contribution of postnatal care, in parallel with antenatal and intrapartum care, as the following example demonstrates:

> The care and support provided for mothers and babies during pregnancy, childbirth and the postnatal period has a significant effect on children's healthy development and their resilience to problems encountered later in life. (p. 6)

and the potential public health impact of high-quality services:

> The quality of the service provided for the half a million babies born in England every year, and their mothers, thus has a long term impact on the future health of the nation. (p. 6)

Recommendations for immediate and ongoing postnatal care were based on a review of the evidence by members of an expert subgroup, with a separate section on maternal mental health. The overriding theme was that postnatal care should be planned with the woman and tailored to meet her individual needs. Changes to the duration of postnatal contacts were recommended, as midwifery discharge at 10–14 days and the end of the postnatal period at 6–8 weeks were viewed as too soon to enable a full assessment of maternal health needs. Midwifery-led services could be provided for at least a month following birth or discharge from hospital and up to three months or longer depending on individual need. The midwives rules and standards published by the Nursing and Midwifery Council in 2004 (NMC 2004) did revise rules with respect to the duration of midwifery care:

> 'Postnatal period' means the period after the end of labour during which the attendance of a midwife upon a mother or baby is required, being not less than ten days and for such a longer period as a midwife considers necessary.

However, Redshaw *et al.* (2007) found only 7% of over 2900 randomly selected women who gave birth in 2006 who returned a questionnaire reported that they received a midwifery visit after 28 days, although this had increased from 2% in 1995 (Garcia *et al.* 1998). Whilst this could infer that there is some flexibility in the system it may also reflect greater needs associated with poorer general health and higher rates of intervention.

NICE guidance for maternity care

The National Institute for Health and Clinical Excellence, established as an independent organisation to assist the NHS in England and Wales to set priorities and make choices, has developed a set of guidelines to inform maternity care and women's health (Box 2.1). Guidance has been developed on specific aspects of NHS practice (i.e. caesarean section, antenatal care) and priority areas to enhance public health (e.g. maternal and infant nutrition). NHS trusts are expected to implement guidance, with compliance assessed by the Care Quality Commission. The challenge of how to support maternity units and staff to integrate NICE maternity service guidance into practice and standards for practice is acknowledged, given the range of national bodies producing guidance including the Royal Colleges, the Confidential Enquiry into Maternal and Child Health and the Health Protection Agency to name but a few. To support implementation of guidelines, NICE produced a range of tools including a costing report and costing template to enable units to calculate costs of implementation, based on their local population.

Box 2.1 NICE guidance relevant to maternity care

- Caesarean section. NICE clinical guideline 13 (2004). Available from: www.nice.org.uk/CG013
- Routine postnatal care of women and their babies. NICE clinical guideline 37 (2006). Available from: www.nice.org.uk/CG037
- Antenatal and postnatal mental health. NICE clinical guideline 45 (2007). Available from: www.nice.org.uk/CG045
- Intrapartum care. NICE clinical guideline 55 (2007). Available from: www.nice.org.uk/CG055
- Antenatal care. NICE clinical guideline 62 (2008). Available from: www.nice.org.uk/CG062
- Diabetes in pregnancy. NICE clinical guideline 63 (2008). Available from: www.nice.org.uk/CG063
- Improving the nutrition of pregnant and breastfeeding mothers and children in low-income households. NICE public health guidance 11 (2008). Available from: www.nice.org.uk/PH011

NICE guidance for postnatal care

As a consequence of increasing evidence that routine postnatal care was not meeting women's needs, the Department of Health and

Welsh Assembly Government commissioned the National Collaborating Centre for Primary Care (NCC-PC) to develop a guideline to inform the routine postnatal care of women and their babies (NICE 2006). The guideline aimed to identify the essential 'core' care all women and their babies should receive in the first 6–8 weeks after birth. Recommendations for practice were based on the best available evidence of clinical and cost-effective care, with guidance included on the following areas:

- Planning the content and delivery of care
- Maternal health
- Infant feeding
- Maintaining infant health

Information and advice to support women to monitor and maintain their own and their baby's health, including the importance of relevant and timely information on a range of health areas are included alongside recommendations for NHS care. The full guideline is available from www.nice.org.uk, with an abridged version for health professionals (Quick Reference Guide) and information for women, their partners or other carers.

Time bands for provision and content of care

NICE (2006) recommends that immediate care (Time Band One) should include taking a woman's blood pressure measurement and ensuring she has passed urine within 6 hours of birth, with action to take if there are concerns. Within 24 hours of the birth, a woman should be offered information on signs and symptoms of major maternal morbidity (see section titled Maternal Morbidity). Time Band Two refers to the content of care between 2 and 7 days post-partum, when women should be offered advice about normal recovery from birth, asked at each contact about their emotional health and well-being, their experience of common health problems and offered support and advice on attachment and positioning to breastfeed and minimise problems such as painful nipples. Management of commonly experienced problems includes 'triggers' for timely and appropriate referral and symptoms identified or reported by the women. Time Band Three covers care and advice provided within 2–6 weeks of the birth. Women should be asked at each contact during this time about their experience of health problems, the timing and resumption of sexual intercourse, resolution of symptoms of transient psychological problems (the blues), with health professionals remaining vigilant to signs of domestic violence. All women should be advised to make an appointment for a final postnatal check at 6–8 weeks.

Planning the content and delivery of care

The guideline recommends that all women have a documented, individualised care plan, which should be developed with the woman as soon as possible after the birth, and ideally commence during the antenatal period. The plan should be based on her previous and current history, taking all relevant factors into account. It is envisaged that by commencing postnatal care planning before the birth, women would feel more prepared and have more appropriate expectations of the impact of birth on their health. The guideline reinforces the recommendation of the NSF (DoH 2004) that each woman has a coordinating health professional, responsible for ensuring she received the right care at the right time. This could be the midwife in the immediate postnatal period, with responsibility passing to the health visitor following midwifery discharge; however, the role could be fulfilled by the most appropriate health professional to meet a woman's needs, including the GP or obstetrician.

Maternal morbidity

The section on maternal health includes guidance on signs and symptoms of major maternal physical morbidity, namely post-partum haemorrhage, pre-eclampsia and eclampsia, thrombosis and genital tract sepsis. A small number of women in the United Kingdom continue to die from these complications in the postnatal period (Lewis 2007) and it is essential that health professionals and women are aware of signs and symptoms of potentially life-threatening conditions to ensure timely referral and management are instigated. As highlighted by the most recent Confidential Enquiry into Maternal and Child Health (CEMACH) report (Lewis 2007), in several cases of maternal death reviewed by the report team, clinical staff did not undertake observations or failed to act promptly on maternal symptoms of pyrexia or tachycardia. Those responsible for providing clinical care after birth, including midwives, GPs, obstetricians and staff in Emergency Departments must be aware of signs and symptoms of acute clinical illness in women after birth. Postnatal management of women who are obese and have a higher risk of thromboembolism should be planned with relevant members of the healthcare team.

Evidence is also presented on commonly experienced maternal morbidity, such as backache, urinary stress incontinence, perineal pain and fatigue, with recommendations for first-line management of these, and an emphasis on the need to ask women at each contact about their experience of morbidity, including their emotional health and well-being. This should include offering women an opportunity to talk about their birth experience and ask questions about their labour and birth. Full guidance on maternal mental health issues is included in a separate NICE guideline on antenatal and postnatal mental health published in 2007 (NICE 2007) and midwives should familiarise themselves with the recommendations presented.

From a midwifery perspective, the NICE postnatal care guidance means that the performance of traditional observations and examinations should not be routinely performed – the emphasis is on asking women about their health and utilising clinical skills more effectively to undertake observation and examination if there is a clinical indication or a woman reports any concerns about her health. With the emphasis on providing women and their families with information and sources of support to assist postnatal recovery, planning of contacts and the content of each contact should be more relevant to meeting the needs of individual women after birth.

Infant feeding

A major issue for public health is the lack of women who do not exclusively breastfeed for the recommended minimum of 6 months given the robust evidence of maternal and infant health benefits that breastfeeding can confer (Renfrew *et al*. 2005). Reasons for early cessation such as painful breasts and insufficient milk continue to be reported (Bolling *et al*. 2007), which suggest poor postnatal support and lack of appropriate follow-up. The infant feeding section of the NICE guideline (NICE 2006) includes information on need for a supportive environment for breastfeeding, with appropriate support regardless of location of care. Breastfed babies should not be given formula feed unless medically indicated and babies should not be separated from their mothers within the first hour of birth unless indicated for the health of the mother or her baby. Advice for women who require additional support to commence and sustain breastfeeding, for example, following caesarean section, is also included. A significant inclusion within the guidance is the recommendation that healthcare facilities have a written breastfeeding policy and an externally evaluated structured programme that encourages breastfeeding, using the Baby Friendly Hospital Initiative as a minimum standard.

Competencies to undertake postnatal care

The postnatal care guideline (NICE 2006) does not refer to which members of the multi-professional team should be responsible for specific postnatal contacts, despite the traditional role of midwives as the main care providers during the first 10–14 days after birth. The guideline instead refers to the level of competency required for a contact, based on criteria included in Skills for Health, the Sector Skills

Council for the UK health sector (www.skillsforhealth.org.uk). In effect, this has paved the way for changes in the skill mix of the health teams responsible for postnatal care, particularly the role of the Maternity Support Worker (MSW) (or Maternity Care Assistant) whose role in postnatal care was referred to in the NSF (DoH 2004). The implications of the introduction of MSWs into postnatal care will be explored more fully in the following section.

This is the first time that national guidance on the level of competency required to undertake postnatal care has been presented, including core competencies which all staff who work with postnatal women should be able to demonstrate. Core competencies include being able to support women to breastfeed, to have an understanding of the physiology of lactation and neonatal metabolic adaptation and ability to communicate this to parents. Competency to undertake maternal and infant examination and recognise abnormalities, to recognise the risks, signs and symptoms of domestic violence and child abuse, including who to contact for advice and management in line with Department of Health guidance, are other core competencies (DoH 2005).

Priorities and challenges facing contemporary postnatal care

The need to improve quality of care and implications of achieving this in line with finite resources continue to be the main drivers impacting on the content of postnatal care and the duration and timing of contacts a woman will receive. As highlighted earlier, although service revision is necessary to meet the needs of women with chronic ill health and complex social needs, barriers to achieving change continue to be presented. 'Maternity Matters' (DoH 2007) outlined the government's commitment to the maternity services in line with an agenda for health reform:

> to develop a patient-led NHS that uses available resources as effectively and fairly as possible to promote health, reduce health inequalities and deliver the best and safest healthcare.

'Maternity Matters' (DoH 2007) proposed that women have a choice of how and where to access postnatal care, which could be in their home or in a community setting, such as a Sure Start Children's Centre, with care delivered and coordinated according to relevant guidelines and an agreed pathway. Publication of 'High Quality Care for All: NHS Next Stage Review Final Report' (DoH 2008) refers to the changes facing society and healthcare systems in the United Kingdom and globally, including increased expectations of service users, the changing nature of disease and changing expectations of the healthcare workforce. This report has implications for commissioning of services, for ongoing quality improvement, education and training of NHS staff. Prior to the launch of the Next Stage Review (DoH 2008), Strategic Health Authorities (SHAs) were asked to develop plans for action. With respect to postnatal services, the NHS London review in line with 'Maternity Matters' (DoH 2007) also referred to women receiving postnatal care at home and/or in a polyclinic. Although mooted as 'choice' in these documents, there is limited information of what this will constitute or how 'choice' will be offered to women, with a dearth of evidence as to the effectiveness of clinic provision for postnatal women. There is also concern that this model may not meet the needs of the most vulnerable women (Bick 2008) and research is urgently required.

Changes to the deployment of the maternity workforces, including the introduction of the European Working Time Directive (NHS Confederation 2004), the reconfiguration of neonatal services, policy drivers and the implementation of NICE maternity guidance are changing the boundaries of professional roles. Both 'Maternity Matters' (DoH 2007) and Health Care for London (NHS London 2007) refer to the key role of maternity support workers in delivering timely and appropriate care. The introduction of MSWs is widespread across the United Kingdom, their role changing from undertaking clerical and physical tasks to providing clinical care (Sandall *et al.* 2007), a change supported by 'Agenda for Change', which modernised pay systems within the NHS to reflect new working practices and skill mix (Woodward *et al.* 2004). To date there has been little information on the role of MSW, their training needs and impact of their introduction on the role of the midwife or maternal and infant health outcomes. Sandall *et al.* (2007) undertook a scoping study on behalf of the Department of Health in England to provide an overview of the number, scope and range of practice, skill mix and service model agreements of MSWs. Findings were based on a structured questionnaire sent to a representative sample of NHS Trusts. Views on pertinent issues were also sought from email list members of an internal and external reference group and all regional Local Supervising Authority midwifery officers.

The researchers found maternity service managers enthusiastic about the contribution of MSWs and the potential for their greater involvement in Sure Start and Children's Centres (Sandall *et al.* 2007). Benefits of the MSW role were highlighted in their support for breastfeeding as they had more time to spend with women, a role which could be provided within the acute and primary care sector. There were some issues with respect to their scope of practice, due to the lack of statutory training or suitability of the National Vocational training, with some MSWs reported to be undertaking tasks such as giving drugs, taking bloods and transferring emergency patients and babies, which would be regarded as midwifery duties. The delegation of duties to a MSW, ensuring midwife compliance with the NMC code of professional conduct, was also identified as an issue, as was the danger that MSW could cease to be 'another pair of hands' on busy labour wards and instead substitute care provided by midwives. With current staffing issues and greater support needs of women who become pregnant facing the UK maternity services, it is likely that the numbers of MSW will increase, however, it is essential that regulation and training of MSWs are addressed as a priority to promote the quality and safety of care. Planned revisions to the place of postnatal care and impact on health outcomes of changes in skill mix of maternity teams should be supported by evidence of benefit rather than as a short-term 'fix' to manage finite resources.

The international perspective

At the end of the first decade of the twenty-first century, access to postnatal care for women in developing countries can still literally mean the difference between life and death for a mother and her baby (Kerber *et al.* 2007). If a mother dies as a result of sepsis or postpartum haemorrhage, there is a high likelihood that her baby will also die. The global HIV/AIDs crisis, epidemics of tuberculosis and spread of diseases such as malaria, further reduce the odds of surviving pregnancy and birth. For women living in areas of civil disturbance and war, these issues are further compounded.

A number of studies from high-middle-and low-income countries are providing evidence of the impact of maternal mortality and morbidity, with increasing recognition of the need for maternal and infant health to be a public health priority, particularly in countries striving to achieve the United Nations Millennium Development Goals (Black *et al.* 2003). Recent studies that have focused on the need to improve services after birth include a planned cluster-randomised trial of a community intervention using local women as facilitators to improve care during pregnancy, birth and the postnatal period in Mumbai, India (Shah More *et al.* 2008), an RCT that compared outcomes among women allocated to receive home visits from specially trained midwives compared with no home visits in Damascus, Syria (Bashour *et al.* 2008) and a Brazilian study that examined the prevalence of postnatal depression among women living in an areas of Southern Brazil (Tannous *et al.* 2008). In some states of the United States of America where women may be offered one postnatal consultation with their doctor at 4–6 weeks after birth, the need to ensure how the most vulnerable women who are least likely to attend their postpartum visit receive the care they need was recently highlighted (Center for Disease Control 2007).

One factor common to all countries which have investigated health outcomes after birth, is the apparent 'invisibility' of the postnatal period and lack of systematic recognition that care in the days and weeks after birth is an essential continuum of pregnancy and birth care (Bick *et al.* 2008). If maternal and infant mortality rates in developing countries are to be reduced in line with the Millennium Development Goals, postnatal care in the hours and days after birth to identify and manage maternal haemorrhage and sepsis are just as essential as ensuring a woman has access to a skilled birth attendant during her labour; if in developed countries such as the United Kingdom, we wish to improve public health outcomes with respect to maternal mental health, improve breastfeeding uptake and duration and tackle chronic health problems caused by the burden of obesity, we need effective postnatal care.

Policy makers and service commissioners and providers should promote and protect postnatal care as an essential component of public health and ensure midwifery and other health service provider skills are optimised to meet health needs in line with national guidance. All women, wherever they give birth in the world, deserve care that will ensure they and their babies have the best start to life. Priorities for maternity services after birth have to be redefined as they are not currently meeting the needs of many women, their babies or families, who have to suffer the longer-term physical and psychological consequences.

Key implications for midwifery practice

- Minimal change has taken place in the organisation and content of midwifery postnatal care since the beginning of the twentieth century, despite significant advances in public health, the dramatic decline in maternal mortality and other changes impacting on women's role in society.
- Evidence of the impact of birth on women's physical and psychological health is accruing. However, much of the evidence is based on short-term outcomes and more research, which also considers longer-term consequences is required.
- Midwives need to be aware of the signs and symptoms of major postnatal morbidity, such as sepsis, thrombosis, post-partum haemorrhage, pre-eclampsia/eclampsia and what immediate action to take if a woman has signs or symptoms indicating serious illness and/or reports feeling unwell. Women and their families also need to be aware of these.
- Midwives also need to be aware of signs and symptoms of more commonly experienced morbidity, such as backache and perineal pain in order that problems can be identified and their impact minimised and women encouraged to discuss health needs with their midwife.

- Social support can make an important contribution to families' well-being and midwives need to ask women about levels of support at each postnatal contact.
- Maternity service commissioners and providers need to ensure postnatal care provision is planned and resourced as a continuum of effective maternity care. Evaluation of postnatal services is essential to ensure provision is in line with NICE maternity guidance and women are receiving the care they need.
- It is also important that midwives and other healthcare staff, including maternity support workers, have the competencies necessary to provide optimal postnatal care for a woman and her baby each at contact.

References

Allen I, Bourke Dowling S, Williams S (1998) *A Leading Role for Midwives? Evaluation of Midwifery Group Practice Development Projects*. Report no. 832. London: Policy Studies Institute.

Audit Commission (1997) *First Class Delivery: Improving Maternity Services in England and Wales*. Abingdon: Audit Commission Publications.

Barrett G, Pendry E, Peacock J, Victor C, Thakar R, Manyonda I (2000) Women's sexual health after childbirth. *British Journal of Obstetrics and Gynaecology* 107: 186–195.

Bashour HN, Kharouf MH, AbdulSalam AA, El Asmar K, Tabbaa MA, Cheika SA (2008) Effect of postnatal home visits on maternal/infant outcomes in Syria: a randomised controlled trial. *Public Health Nursing* 25 (2): 115–125.

Bick D (2008) The conundrum of maternity service policy for postnatal care. *Midwives*: 42–43.

Bick D, Bastos MH, Diniz S (2008, in press) Unlocking the potential of effective care for life-long maternal and infant health: the need to address the 'invisible' service after birth. *Latin American Journal of Nursing (Revista Latin-Americana de Enfermagem)* 42 (3): 416–421.

Bick D, MacArthur C (1995a) The extent, severity and effect of health problems after childbirth. *British Journal of Midwifery* 3 (1): 27–31.

Bick D, MacArthur C (1995b) Attendance, content and relevance of the 6 week postnatal examination. *Midwifery* 11: 69–73.

Black R, Morris S, Bryce J (2003) Child survival 1. Where and why are 10 million children dying every year? *Lancet* 361: 2226–2234.

Bolling K, Grant C, Hamlyn B, Thornton A (2007) *Infant Feeding Survey 2005*. London: The Information Centre.

Brown S, Lumley J (1998) Maternal health after childbirth: results of an Australian population based survey. *British Journal of Obstetrics and Gynaecology* 105: 156–161.

Center for Disease Control (2007) Postpartum care visits – 11 States and New York City, 2004. *Morbidity and Mortality Weekly Report* 56 (50): 1312–1316.

Cox JL, Holden JM, Sagovsky R (1987) Detection of postnatal depression. Development of the 10-item Edinburgh postnatal depression scale. *British Journal of Psychiatry* 150: 782–786.

Department of Health (1993) *Changing Childbirth: The Report of the Expert Maternity Committee.* London: The Stationery Office.

Department of Health (1999) *Saving Lives: Our Healthier Nation.* London: The Stationery Office.

Department of Health (2000) *The NHS Plan; A Plan for Investment, A Plan for Reform.* London: The Stationery Office.

Department of Health (2004) *National Service Framework for Children, Young People and Maternity Services.* London: The Stationery Office.

Department of Health (2005) *Responding to Domestic Abuse: A Handbook for Health Professionals.* London: Department of Health. Available at: www.dh.gov.uk.

Department of Health (2007) *Partnerships for Children, Families and Maternity. Maternity Matters: Choice, Access and Continuity of Care in a Safe Service.* Available at: www.dh.gov.uk.

Department of Health (2008) *High Quality Care for All: NHS Next Stage Final Review.* Available at: www.doh.gov.uk.

Garcia J, Redshaw M, Fitzsimons B, Keene K (1998) *First Class Delivery: A National Survey of Women's Views of Maternity Care.* London: Audit Commission.

Garcia J, Renfrew M, Marchant S (1994) Postnatal home visiting by midwives. *Midwifery* 10: 40–43.

Glazener C (1997) Sexual function after childbirth: women's experiences, persistent morbidity and lack of professional recognition. *British Journal of Obstetrics and Gynaecology* 104: 330–335.

Glazener C, Abdalla M, Stroud P, Templeton A, Russell I (1995) Postnatal maternal morbidity: extent, causes, prevention and treatment. *British Journal of Obstetrics and Gynaecology* 102: 282–287.

Gunn J, Lumley J, Chondros P, Young D (1998) Does an early postnatal check-up improve maternal health: results from a randomised trial in Australian general practice. *British Journal of Obstetrics and Gynaecology* 105: 991–997.

House of Commons Select Committee (1992) *Winterton Report.* London: The Stationery Office.

Hunter B (2007) *The All Wales Clinical Pathway for Normal Labour: What are the Experiences of Midwives, Doctors, Managers and Mothers?* Final Project Report. The Health Foundation.

Kerber KJ, de Graft-Johnson JE, Bhutta ZA, Okong P, Starrs A, Lawn J (2007) Continuum of care for maternal, newborn, and child health: from slogan to service delivery. *Lancet* 370: 1358–1369.

King's Fund (2005) *An Independent Audit of the NHS UNDER LABOUR 1997–2005.* London: King's Fund.

Lewis G (2007) The Confidential Enquiry into Maternal and Child Health (CEMACH) Saving mothers' lives: reviewing maternal deaths to make motherhood safer 2003 to 2005. *The Seventh Report of the Confidential Enquiries into Maternal Deaths in the United Kingdom.* London: CEMACH.

MacArthur C (1999) What does postnatal care do for women's health? *Lancet* 353 (9150): 343–344.

MacArthur C, Glazener C, Lancashire R, Herbison P, Wilson D, Grant A (2005) Faecal Incontinence and mode of first and subsequent delivery: a six year longitudinal study. *British Journal of Obstetrics and Gynaecology* 112 (8): 1075–1082.

MacArthur C, Lewis M, Knox E (1991) *Health After Childbirth*. London: HMSO.

MacArthur C, Winter H, Bick D, *et al.* (2002) Effects of redesigned community postnatal care on women's health 4 months after birth: a cluster randomised controlled trial. *Lancet* 359: 378–385.

MacArthur C, Winter HR, Bick DE, *et al.* (2003) *Redesigning Post Natal Care; A Randomised Controlled Trial of Protocol Based, Midwifery Led Care Focused on Individual Women's Physical and Psychological Health Needs*. NHS R&D, NCC HTA.

Mander R, Smith G (2008) Saving Mothers' Lives (formerly Why Mothers die): reviewing maternal deaths to make motherhood safer 2003–2005. *Midwifery* 24 (1): 8–12.

Maynard A, Street A (2006) Seven years of feast, seven years of famine: boom to bust in the NHS? *British Medical Journal* 332: 906–908.

Morrell C, Spiby H, Stewart P, Walters S, Morgan A (2000) Costs and effectiveness of community postnatal support workers: randomised controlled trial. *British Medical Journal* 321: 593–598.

Murphy-Black T (1989) *Postnatal Care at Home: A Descriptive Study of Mother's Needs and the Maternity Services*. Edinburgh: University of Edinburgh Nursing Research Unit.

National Institute for Health and Clinical Excellence (2006) *Routine Postnatal Care of Women and their Babies. Clinical Guideline 37*.

National Institute for Health and Clinical Excellence (2007) *Antenatal and Postnatal Mental Health. Clinical Guideline 45*.

NHS Confederation (2004) *Future Healthcare Network Survey of Models of Maternity Care: Towards Sustainable WTD Compliant Staffing and Clinical Network Solutions*, www.nhsconfed.org.uk (accessed 11/11/2008).

NHS London (2007) *Healthcare for London: A Framework for Action*. London: NHS London.

Nursing and Midwifery Council (2004) *Midwives Rules and Standards*. London: NMC.

Redshaw M, Rowe R, Hockley C, Brocklehurst P (2007) *Recorded Delivery: A National Survey of Women's Experience of Maternity Care 2006*. Oxford: National Perinatal Epidemiology Unit, University of Oxford.

Reid M, Glazener C, Murray G, Taylor G (2002) A twocentred pragmatic randomised controlled trial of two interventions of postnatal support. *British Journal of Obstetrics and Gynaecology* 109: 1164–1170.

Renfrew M, Dyson L, Wallace L, D'Souza L, McCormick F, Spiby H (2005) *The Effectiveness of Public Health Interventions to Promote the Duration of Breastfeeding Systematic Review*, 1st Edition. National Institute for Health and Clinical Excellence.

Richardson A, Mmata C (2007) *NHS Maternity Statistics England 2005–2006.* London: The Information Centre.

Rycroft-Malone J, Fontenla M, Bick D, Seers K (2008) Protocol based care: impact on roles and service delivery. *Journal of Evaluation of Clinical Practice* 14 (5): 867–873.

Sandall J, Manthorpe J, Mansfield A, Spencer L (2007) *Support Workers in Maternity Services: A National Scoping Study of NHS Trusts Providing Maternity Care in England 2006.* London: King's College London.

Saurel-Cubizolles M-J, Romito P, Lelong N, Ancel P-Y (2000) Women's health after childbirth: a longitudinal study in France and Italy. *British Journal of Obstetrics and Gynaecology* 107: 1202–1209.

Shah More N, Bapat U, Das S, *et al.* (2008) *Cluster-Randomised Controlled Trial of Community Mobilisation in Mumbai Slums to Improve Care During Pregnancy, Delivery, Postpartum and for the Newborn.* Study protocol. BMC Trials, http://www.trialsjournal.com/contents/9/1/7.

Sharif K, Clarke P, Whittle M (1993) Routine six weeks postnatal examination: to do or not to do? *Journal of Obstetrics and Gynaecology* 4 (13): 251–252.

Shields N, Reid M, Cheyne H, *et al.* (1997) Impact of midwife managed care in the postnatal period: an exploration of psychosocial outcomes. *Journal of Reproductive and Infant Psychology* 15: 91–108.

Tannous L, Gigante LP, Fuchs SC, Busnello EDA (2008) Postnatal depression in Southern Brazil: prevalence and its demographic and socioeconomic determinants. *BMC Psychiatry*, http://www.biomedcentral.com/1471-244X/8/1.

Tew M (1998) *Safer Childbirth: A Critical History of Maternity Care.* London: Free Association Books Ltd.

Thew M, Paech MJ (2007) Management of postdural puncture headache in the obstetric patient. *Current Opinion in Anesthesiology* 21 (3): 288–292.

Turnbull D, Holmes A, Shields N, *et al.* (1996) Randomised, controlled trial of efficacy of midwife-managed care. *Lancet* 348: 213–218.

United Kingdom Central Council for Nursing Midwives and Health Visitors (1998) *Midwives' Rules and Code of Practice.* London: UKCC.

Woodward V, Clawson L, Ineichen B (2004) Maternity support workers: what is their role? *Midwives* 7 (9): 390–393.

Chapter 3
Women's and Midwives' Views of Early Postnatal Care

Jane Yelland

Introduction

A statement made by the UK Audit Commission over a decade ago still rings true today:

> There is some uncertainty about what postnatal care is aiming to achieve – whether it is solely to prevent and treat immediate health problems in the mother and the baby or whether it is aiming to enhance the overall experience, giving mothers time to recover and get to know her baby ... perhaps because of this uncertainty there is considerable variation in the nature of postnatal care ...
>
> (UK Audit Commission 1997)

There remains uncertainty among both providers and recipients of postnatal care as to what constitutes appropriate care in the time following birth. The absence in some agencies and diversity among others, of principals and objectives guiding postnatal care make it difficult to know how maternity facilities and postnatal services approach service delivery in this area. Listening to women's and midwives' views provides valuable information about the organisation and provision of postnatal care.

The literature indicates that it is this aspect of childbirth that receives little attention, with a dearth of papers regarding women's and midwives' views of postnatal care. Indeed postnatal care is occasionally dubbed the 'poor cousin' or the 'Cinderella' of maternity care when considered against the emphasis placed on the antenatal or intrapartum periods.

This chapter examines the small body of literature on the views and experiences of postnatal care both from a consumer perspective and from the providers of care, predominantly midwives. For the purposes of this chapter, the focus is on the very early postnatal period, which could be loosely defined as the first week or two following birth.

Most of the studies of postnatal care are from developed countries where women generally spend some days in hospital following the birth. Some go on to have the option of receiving care at home following discharge. Diversity in terms of the length of the postnatal hospital stay, arrangements for home-based visits and the involvement of other maternal and child health services in the early postnatal period limits comparisons between countries such as Australia, Canada, the United States, the United Kingdom and countries of western Europe. Yet findings from recent studies identify many similarities in terms of women's experiences and midwives' views and it is these similarities within the context of diversity that are discussed in the following text.

Assessing women's views and experiences

Patient satisfaction with the health care and the health services that people receive is of growing interest. This interest is illustrated by the extensive health-related literature over the past three decades (Crow *et al.* 2002). Maternity care with its more 'consumer' orientation has increasingly been the focus of satisfaction studies (Sullivan *et al.* 1982; Lumley 1985; Bramadat *et al.* 1993; Christiaens *et al.* 2007).

Defining and measuring patient satisfaction is difficult (Carr-Hill 1992; Bramadat *et al.* 1993; Sitzia *et al.* 1997) and conceptually it is impossible to derive an objective measure of satisfaction. Ratings of satisfaction have been shown to vary according to where the assessment takes place, when the assessment occurs, who undertakes the assessment and how the assessments are made (Lumley 1985; Jacoby *et al.* 1990). 'Satisfaction' with care is a multidimensional concept requiring an appreciation of the multitude of expectations and experiences that contribute to a satisfaction rating. High ratings of satisfaction in relation to a global question often underestimates the level of dissatisfaction with specific aspects of care (Locker *et al.* 1978; Brown *et al.* 1997).

In acknowledging the complexity of maternity care, deconstructing satisfaction and hearing women's views of what contributes to their experience of care is important – important as it provides an indication of the quality of the care provided; important as it should shape future policy, planning and practice.

There are other reasons why women's views and experiences matter and they relate to women themselves. Garcia (1999) argues that women's views matter because women's reactions to care in pregnancy and postnatally can affect the way they care for themselves and their babies and their future help-seeking behaviour.

Studies that examine women's views and experiences of postnatal care have used a variety of methods, primarily cross-sectional survey design or qualitative methods including interviews and focus groups. Predominantly, studies have examined the experiences of women throughout the entire childbirth experience, incorporating questions related to postnatal care. Very few have explored postnatal care explicitly. Those that have identify some methodological constraints. Many draw conclusions from small sample sizes, with participants selected from one or two agencies, and hence acknowledge problems related to generalisability of the findings.

Ratings of care

Quantitative information on women's views of care is often collected via questions using scales (ratings of 'very satisfied' to 'very dissatisfied' or 'very good' to 'very poor'). In several studies, an *a priori* decision has been taken to classify responses of less than 'very satisfied' or less than 'very good' as indicating a level of dissatisfaction or that some aspect of care could have been better (Carr-Hill 1992).

Overall how do women rate the hospital care they receive following birth?

In most developed countries, women give birth in hospitals and are cared for there for a varying length of time following the birth. The time women spend in hospital following birth has declined gradually over recent decades, not always with a corresponding shift to early postnatal care being provided at home.

While only a few studies of satisfaction with maternity care have examined women's views of hospital postnatal care explicitly, those that have report strikingly consistent findings. The 1990s saw some of the first population-based data on women's experiences of maternity care including the early post-partum period.

In the United Kingdom, the national survey of women who had recently given birth conducted by the Audit Commission 10 years ago reported relatively poor ratings of postnatal hospital care (Garcia 1998) with differences between women's expectations of the help that they would get for themselves and the baby in the postnatal ward and what they actually received. Participants responding to questions about what constitutes particularly good care frequently mentioned being treated as an individual and the importance of the kindness and concern of caregivers.

When the UK national survey was repeated in 2006, women were again more critical of postnatal hospital care than the care received during pregnancy and labour and birth. The value of individualised care was recognised by survey participants. During the hospital stay only half of the women felt that they were treated as individuals by the staff, with 1 in 10 women reporting that they were never or rarely treated in this way (Redshaw *et al.* 2007).

In 1994, a population-based survey of recent mothers was conducted in the state of Victoria, Australia. A postal survey 6 months following the birth (Brown *et al.* 1997) asked women to give an overall rating of their care during the antenatal period, during labour and birth and during the postnatal hospital stay. The survey was repeated in 2000 with a larger sample. Consistent and striking findings from these surveys were the poor overall ratings of hospital postnatal care. Only 52% (685/1325) of women in 1994 and 51% (814/1602) in 2000 described their postnatal care in hospital as 'very good' (Brown *et al.* 2005). This contrasts with significantly higher overall ratings of antenatal and intrapartum care (Bruinsma *et al.* 2003).

The strongest association with negative ratings of care were related to women's experiences of specific aspects of care, especially the perceived quality of their interactions with care providers (further discussed on page 54). Other factors associated with satisfaction were geographic locality (rural/metropolitan), private admission status and country of birth (Darcy *et al.* 2001).

The Swedish study of maternal satisfaction with maternity care identified that the characteristics of women were associated with their assessment of care (Waldenstrom *et al.* 2006). Parity was not associated with satisfaction. Single women were less likely to rate their postnatal hospital care highly, with the authors suggesting that women who experience little or no support from their partner may feel lonely or abandoned in a hospital environment where the presence of the baby's father is common practice.

In a complementary study to the Victorian Survey of Recent Mothers 1994, migrant women of non-English-speaking background were interviewed about their views and experiences of maternity care. The largely representative group of Filipino, Turkish and Vietnamese women participating in the study rated their postnatal hospital stay very poorly. These women indicated that the need for rest, access to interpreting support and care providers' enquiry about preferences (e.g. cultural) are paramount to what constitutes quality postnatal care (Yelland *et al.* 1998).

Waldenstrom *et al.* (2006) investigated satisfaction with intrapartum and hospital post-partum care in a national sample of 4600 Swedish-speaking women, surveyed at 2 and 12 months following the birth. When the outcome variables were dichotomized into women who were satisfied ('very positive' or 'positive') with care and those that were not or had mixed feelings, 26% of participants fell into the 'dissatisfied' category. Further analysis was based on this dichotomy. However, a different picture of satisfaction emerges taking the most positive rating of care. Only 35% of women participating in the Swedish study gave a 'very positive' assessment of their post-partum care – indicating that three-quarters of women were dissatisfied with aspect/s of their care. As other studies have reported, overall assessment of intrapartum care was higher than that of postnatal care.

While it is difficult to make comparisons when the questions and approach to analysis differs, it is clear from this Swedish study and the UK and Australian surveys that hospital postnatal care is not viewed or experienced favourably by a significant number of women.

It has been argued that reorganising service delivery to promote continuity of caregiver may enhance individualised care and satisfaction with the postnatal period. Yet, findings from the trials of team midwifery care also report lower levels of satisfaction with postnatal hospital care than with any other episode of care (Waldenström *et al.* 2000; Homer *et al.* 2002a; Biro *et al.* 2003). It is often postnatal care that remains the least altered in the introduction of a new model, given that the postnatal unit is the only option for accommodating and caring for women following birth, irrespective of the model attended.

Exceptions to this reinforce the idea that a philosophy and the delivery of individualised care can make a difference. Women who attended midwife-run birth centres and participated in the Australian survey of recent mothers in the 1990s were significantly more likely to rate their postnatal care as 'very good' compared to women in other public models of care and women attending private obstetrician-led care (Brown & Lumley 1998). Midwife care in these centres involved a small group of midwives caring for women through each episode of care, within a common philosophy and in a discrete unit within a hospital setting.

The randomised controlled trial (RCT) of the efficacy of midwife-managed care in Glasgow over a decade ago (Turnbull *et al.* 1996) provides evidence that the organisation of care and the ability to promote continuity of care through the postnatal period is an important element in improving women's satisfaction with care after birth. The trial group in the Turnbull study was cared for by a named midwife with backup from a team of midwives through each of the three episodes of care, including care received in hospital following the birth. Women in the midwife care group were more likely to be pleased with their post-partum experience and significantly more likely to be satisfied with information, decision-making and individualised care than women in the standard care group.

A UK pilot project evaluating satisfaction and clinical outcomes for two groups of women cared for by either a team of midwives or in a traditional model of care (Hicks *et al.* 2003) reported that the experimental group were significantly more satisfied with several aspects of postnatal care including having their views taken into account, sensitivity of staff, explanations and consultation and consistency of information.

The body of evidence that emerged in the 1990s in relation to continuity of care provided impetus for a group of hospitals in Australia to reform the organisation and provision of maternity care. Over a 2-year period a major change was introduced including the reorganisation of midwifery staffing, the introduction of evidence-based guidelines (e.g. breastfeeding), new consumer-written information, the introduction of postnatal planning visits in pregnancy and the establishment of hospital-based domiciliary service. An evaluation of these changes indicated a small but significant improvement in women's ratings of postnatal hospital care; the level of advice and support received in relation to discharge and going home; and the sensitivity of caregivers (Yelland *et al.* 2009).

What aspects of postnatal care are important to women?

There are limitations with global ratings, which lack sensitivity to specific aspects of care. The population-based surveys of recent mothers discussed earlier and smaller descriptive studies (e.g. Woollett *et al.* 1990; Stamp *et al.* 1994; Murray *et al.* 2000; Forster *et al.* 2008) have included questions and invited open-ended comments in relation to aspects of care. An examination of specific areas of care provides clues as to what contributes to women's overall ratings and satisfaction with care and what reform or interventions are likely to make a difference.

Rudman *et al.* (2007) investigated individual variation in the experiences of 2338 women of different aspects of postnatal hospital care and identified a more varied and negative picture of women's experiences compared with studies based on a single item of overall care. Examination of women's appraisal of four different aspects of care including interpersonal care, time spent on physical checks, time spent on information and support and time spent on assistance with breastfeeding revealed that women are not necessarily either 'satisfied' or 'dissatisfied' in a general sense, but with one or more of these aspects. Clusters of women were identified according to their satisfaction with each aspect of care, with further analysis revealing that these clusters were related to maternal characteristics, labour outcomes and the way in which postnatal care was organised. Rudman and colleagues concluded that care needs to be individualised, with the carer taking into account an understanding of the domains of what contributes to a satisfying and health-enhancing experience.

Some of these domains and factors that impact on women's rating of their postnatal care are covered under four broad themes: spending time in hospital following birth; home visiting following discharge; interactions and communication with care providers; and continuity and consistency of care.

The hospital stay

The most obvious and dramatic change in early postnatal care in developed countries is the reduction in the length of time women spend in hospital following birth. Yet despite this significant shift in the organisation of care, little evidence exists as to the impact of earlier discharge on maternal and infant health, or women's views of care associated with varying length of hospital stay or alternative community-based options for early postnatal care.

A recently updated Cochrane review of early postnatal discharge from hospital for healthy mothers and term infants included 10 trials and 4489 women. The authors, Brown and colleagues, noted that the findings were inconclusive:

> Methodological limitations of included trials mean that some caution is required in drawing conclusions based on pooled estimates. There were no significant differences between the groups for any outcomes ... It remains unclear how important home midwifery or nursing support is to the safety and acceptability of early discharge programs.
>
> (Brown *et al.* 2009)

The reviewers concluded that policies of earlier postnatal discharge of healthy mothers and term infants do not appear to have adverse effects on breastfeeding or maternal depression when accompanied by a policy of offering women at least one nurse–midwife home visit post discharge. Their concluding comment remains the same as the one made in the original review of 2004 (Brown *et al.* 2004b) that there continues to be a need for large well-designed trials of early discharge programs to inform practice.

In the Swedish study included in the Cochrane review (Waldenstrom & Lindmark *et al.* 1987), women randomised to early discharge were significantly less likely to report dissatisfaction with their postnatal hospital care (14/50 versus 47/54, RR = 0.33 [0.20–0.51]). The three trials that report data on satisfaction in the form of mean scores all found greater satisfaction with postnatal care among women randomised to early discharge (Carty & Bradley *et al.* 1990; Brooten *et al.* 1994; Gagnon *et al.* 1997).

A randomised controlled trial conducted in Switzerland (Boulvain *et al.* 2004) reported that early discharge from hospital supported by midwifery home visits was an acceptable form of care. However, the trial was stopped early due to financial constraints and was subsequently underpowered to assess differences in their main outcome measure, including women's views of care.

In the absence of large and well-designed trials, observational studies provide the next layer of evidence regarding outcomes and women's experiences of varying lengths of stay. In the 2000 population-based survey of recent mothers in Victoria, Australia, the length of the hospital stay following birth was one of the factors associated with satisfaction with postnatal care. Staying in hospital for 1–2 days was associated with less positive ratings of care than a stay of 5 days or more (Brown *et al.* 2005). Waldenstrom *et al.* (2006), in a national study of satisfaction with intrapartum and postnatal care, noted that maternal or infant health problems, which motivated a longer length of hospital stay, had a greater impact on women's overall assessment of care than the duration of postnatal care as such.

When data from the three Victorian surveys (conducted in 1989, 1994 and 2000) was compared, Brown *et al.* (2004a) concluded that a shorter length of stay did not appear to have an adverse impact on breastfeeding or women's emotional well-being.

Another Australian study examined the feasibility of introducing new options for postnatal care including 'packages' of shorter length of hospital stay with increased midwife home visits and/or continuity of midwife carer (Forster *et al.* 2007). Participating women reported that they wanted to stay in hospital until they were confident of looking after their babies at home. There was a perception that being in hospital to learn skills related to breastfeeding and the care of their new babies would increase their confidence, especially among first-time mothers. An additional factor is that women in this study viewed the hospital as the 'safe' alternative for care after birth with access to midwifery support and emergency medical intervention 24 hours/day.

Some of the participants in the focus group study experienced post-natal care that they considered inadequate. The quality of professional care, inconsistent advice and a lack of encouragement of the involve-ment of their partner were raised. However, negative experiences or perceived deficiencies in care did not result in women wanting to leave hospital earlier (Forster *et al.* 2008).

Over two decades have passed since Porter and Macintyre (1984) published 'What is, must be best' in which they remarked that

> Women tend to assume that whatever system of care is provided has been well thought-out and therefore likely to be the best one. Where they express a preference, it is generally for whatever arrangements they have experienced than for other possible arrangements. (p. 1197)

It seems that in relation to early postnatal care this still rings true today. While women are critical of many aspects of their postnatal care, they are reluctant to consider alternative options, particularly spending less time in hospital following the birth.

Home visiting following discharge

Domiciliary and home-visiting programs following hospital discharge only exist in a handful of countries and vary widely in terms of universality, the organisation and provision of care and the professional background of the provider. Strikingly, little attention has been given to hearing women's views of early postnatal home visiting. Evaluations of these programs in terms of maternal and infant outcomes and satisfaction with care are sparse. Of all the RCTs of early discharge, none included separate measures of women's views about the availability or quality of postnatal care following discharge.

The United Kingdom has a long history of postnatal home visiting, traditionally provided by health visitors. The role of the health visitor has changed over time, with an increasing focus on screening, surveillance, immunisation and child protection (Billingham & Hall 1998). As health visitors provide care following discharge from midwifery care and can visit a woman and her family until the child commences school, evaluation of this service has often focused on child health outcomes rather than maternal and early infancy outcomes.

A three-arm RCT conducted in the United Kingdom aimed to assess whether increased postnatal support would impact on maternal and infant outcomes for women living in disadvantaged city areas (Wiggins *et al.* 2004). Standard home visiting was compared with home visits by a support health visitor (SHV) where the focus was on listening and exploring issues women wanted to discuss. In the third arm of the trial, support was offered by local community group support (CGS). At the 12- and 18-month follow-up points, there were no significant differences for any of the primary outcomes (child injury, maternal smoking and maternal psychological well-being). There were differences in secondary outcomes: reduced use of general practitioner services for the infants in the SHV group but increased use of health visitor and social worker services, compared to the standard care group. SHV mothers were less worried about their child's health and development, and satisfaction with the intervention among this group was high. However, it should be noted that uptake of the community intervention was low (19%) compared with 94% for the health visitor support program.

In a large RCT in the United Kingdom, where postnatal community-based care was redesigned to provide enhanced midwifery home-visits with care tailored to meet the needs of women, women's mental health measures were significantly better in the intervention group than the control group at 4 months and 12 months post-partum (MacArthur *et al.* 2002, 2003). The authors concluded that redesigned postnatal care with a focus on midwife-led and flexible care could help to improve women's mental health and reduce probable depression at 4 months post-partum.

Traditionally there has been no post-partum follow-up of new mothers in the United States, with the exception of the 6-week check. Various alternatives have been trialled, including postnatal care centres and community-based breastfeeding centres.

In an early postnatal discharge study conducted in the United States, low-risk women were randomised to postnatal home visits or hospital-based group follow-up visits following a hospital stay of 48 hours or less (Escobar *et al.* 2001). Care at home focused on maternal and infant health including physical checks. Hospital-based group care focused primarily on infant care and breastfeeding problems. Telephone interviews with women 2 weeks following discharge showed that there were no significant differences in newborn or maternal readmissions, breastfeeding rates and maternal depressive symptoms. The home visits were more costly but were associated with higher maternal satisfaction. Women in the home-care group were much more likely to rate aspects of care highly compared to the hospital-based group including convenience; the amount of time caregivers spent with them; the caring attitude of the provider and the advice given.

In Canada, post-partum follow-up is provided most frequently by public health nurses in the form of home visits. A Canadian study (Steel O'Connor *et al.* 2003) investigated alternative forms of postnatal public health nurse care following early discharge from hospital. Women were randomised to two home visits (one on the first working day following discharge and another at 10 days post-partum) or a screening telephone call by the public health nurse. The telephone call was structured to elicit a mother's concerns in terms of infant feeding, her baby's general health and her emotional health status. No differences were detected between the groups in maternal confidence, health problems of infants or rates of breastfeeding at 6 months. Around one-third of women in the home visit group refused a visit. Unfortunately, no account is given of women's views of an early postnatal 'screening' telephone call or home visits.

There are methodological limitations with these studies including small sample sizes, lack of statistical power, uptake of the intervention and the validity of outcome measures. Women's views of, and satisfaction with, alternative options for home-based care were not specified primary outcomes. These studies cannot be compared because of these limitations, differences in methodology and differences in primary outcome measures. Their generalisability is also limited given the risk status of those included and the context in which postnatal care was provided.

These studies, however, do suggest that one significant factor – individualised care – is a factor that is paramount to quality care irrespective of *where* care is provided. Care that is more individualised in meeting the needs of each woman is more highly valued than care that is structured, regimented and lacks flexibility in the way that it is provided.

Women's experiences of caregivers

A dominant theme from the literature is the strong association between satisfaction with postnatal care and women's experiences of the people who cared for them. While some studies identify the physical surroundings of postnatal wards, the standard of accommodation, the impact of visitors, noise and interruptions as having an impact on how women view their experience, most report that caregivers and the care they provide is the salient factor in terms of women's satisfaction.

Surveys of recent mothers indicate the importance of the relationship and interactions with caregivers as being associated with more positive experiences of postnatal care (Garcia *et al.* 1998; Proctor 1998; Yelland *et al.* 1998; Green *et al.* 1990, 2000; Small *et al.* 1999; Homer *et al.* 2002a). Brown *et al.* indicated that women were much more likely to be happy with their care when caregivers are sensitive and understanding; take time and are not rushed; and provide helpful advice and support (Brown *et al.* 2005).

This is also evident in several studies examining the views and experiences of migrant women. It is commonly believed that culturally women want to adhere to traditional practices following birth and that the organisation of care should allow this to occur. Yet, the first Australian survey of a largely representative group of migrant women conducted in Victoria found that this was not the case. Turkish, Filipino and Vietnamese women participating in the Mothers in a New Country study were far less concerned about the fact that caregivers knew little about their cultural practices, and more concerned about the care they experienced as unkind and unsupportive. It was the relationship with caregivers and the extent to which women encountered care that was kind, sympathetic and friendly that coloured their experience (Small *et al.* 1997).

This is not to underestimate the contribution that language and communication problems make to how migrant women experience care. Women with low levels of fluency in English reported more problems in communicating with health professionals, resulting in a far less positive experience of care (Small *et al.* 1999).

A small number of studies have explored immigrant women's views of maternity care in detail. Several focus on specific aspects of care particularly related to postnatal issues including infant feeding (Fishman *et al.* 1988; Homer *et al.* 2002b; McLachlan *et al.* 2006) and maternal and infant health (Rice 1999) and early postnatal care (Stamp *et al.* 1994; Tran *et al.* 2001). An interview study of Asian women in East London (Woollett *et al.* 1990) examined postnatal hospital care, identifying differing expectations between woman and their caregivers in relation to responsibility for baby care and the need for rest following birth. This British study, a US study (Lazarus *et al.* 1990) and Australian studies (Cape 1999; Small *et al.* 1999) have all suggested that immigrant women's dissatisfaction with care is linked to quality of care issues rather than the role of culture.

Many of these studies indicate that positive interactions lead to health professionals engaging with women as individuals and with respect for individual circumstances, preferences and needs. Lauver *et al.* suggests that the 'content' of individualised care develops from the interaction between patient and care provider (Lauver *et al.* 2002). The finding that only half of the women participating in the last national survey in the United Kingdom reported that they were 'always' treated as individuals during their postnatal hospital stay (Redshaw *et al.* 2007) provides renewed pressure to restructure care to one that focuses on the individual rather than on women's assumed needs, and with a move away from care that is provided in a structured and predetermined way.

Continuity and consistency of care

Midwifery textbooks state that the aim of postnatal care is to monitor and promote the health of the mother and baby and assist with lactation and education in relation to the care of the infant (Marchant 2003; Bick 2004). The provision of education and advice is a theme of the UK NICE (National Institute for Health and Clinical Excellence) postnatal care guidelines.

The promotion of breastfeeding has dominated the literature in terms of the provision of education and advice in the postnatal period. In the statewide review of postnatal care in Australia, care providers interviewed identified the provision of information and advice as one of the main aims of postnatal care with a strong sense that the postnatal period was a time for education of women – primarily in caring for their babies including infant feeding (Forster *et al.* 2005).

Women's unhappiness about conflicting advice emerged in some of the very early studies of maternity care (i.e. Oakley 1979), continued to be raised in research conducted in the following years (i.e. Green *et al.* 1988) and remains a persistent source of concern among mothers in more recent studies of maternity care (i.e. Garcia *et al.* 1998). Conflicting advice and the problems that this can cause for women is often related to the advice and information given regarding breastfeeding.

There is a strong link between consistency of the provision of information and advice and continuity of care, primarily the caregiver. With such diversity in the organisation and provision of maternity care and less of an opportunity for women to have continuity of caregiver during this episode of care, it is hardly surprising that women often comment on receiving inconsistent or conflicting information and advice during the postnatal period.

Maternity care in many countries remains fragmented. Arguably fragmentation is at its greatest during the early postnatal period where hospital midwives, domiciliary midwives, home-visiting health professionals, maternal and child health services and general practitioners have a part to play in the provision of care. Postnatal care, particularly care provided in hospital, is also the most difficult episode of care to reorientate in order to offer continuity of caregiver.

The expansion of primary midwifery models of care including birth centre team midwifery, midwifery group practice and caseload midwifery, with a focus on continuity of care/carer through each episode of care including the early postnatal period, aims to improve maternal and infant outcomes and enhance women's experiences of care. Evaluation of previous programs suggests that continuity of caregiver by midwife teams or a primary midwife is likely to show beneficial effects, particularly in terms of information, advice and maternal satisfaction (Flint *et al.* 1989; Rowley *et al.* 1995; Turnbull *et al.* 1996), with some evidence of reduced intervention in labour and birth (Harvey *et al.* 1996; Waldenström *et al.* 1998; Homer *et al.* 2002a). A trial of caseload midwifery currently underway in Melbourne, Australia, will examine a number of maternal outcomes including postnatal depression, breastfeeding duration and satisfaction with care (McLachlan *et al.* 2008).

Green *et al.* (2000) reviewed seven UK studies of continuity of midwife care, concluding that none of the studies suggests that women value continuity for its own sake; rather women value what they expect to follow from continuity, that is, consistent care from someone they can trust. It is this consistency of care and the quality of the interactions with caregivers that women appear to value most (Brown *et al*. 2005).

Midwives' views

Studies examining midwives' views of postnatal care are predominantly confined to those undertaken in the United Kingdom and Australia. It is interesting to note that while increasing attention is given to examining consumer's views, experiences and satisfaction with care, far less attention is given to the views and opinions of those who provide that care.

A small exploratory study of midwives' views of hospital and home-based postnatal care in a UK teaching hospital (Catrell *et al*. 2005) identified that midwives felt that they could not always provide optimal care. The study found that midwives considered that the priorities for postnatal care included providing women with physical and emotional support after birth and the provision of parenting information; that societal expectations of motherhood influenced women's views, yet social support was often lacking and that midwives were most satisfied with the provision of postnatal care when their work involved providing individualised care and continuity. Barriers to providing postnatal care were identified, including spending time on administrative duties and a lack of staff.

Similar organisational and resource pressures were noted in a study exploring the quality of the interactions between midwives and women in relation to breastfeeding (Dykes 2005). These pressures, including a perception that postnatal care requires less staff than other episodes of maternity care and the constant movement of staff out of postnatal wards to assist in other areas, resulted in midwives feeling that they had less opportunity or time to establish relationships with women in order to meet their needs.

Proctor (1998) conducted focus groups to compare women's and midwives' perceptions of maternity care. Women's main concerns in the postnatal period focused on the need for information and in developing confidence in knowledge and ability to adjust to the new role of mother. Few participating midwives spoke of the aspects of care that mattered to these women, with the exception of support for breastfeeding.

In an Australian review of public hospital postnatal care, data was collected via a postal questionnaire to all hospitals with maternity facilities in the state of Victoria and by interview with randomly selected midwife key informants (Forster *et al*. 2005).

The midwives participating in the postnatal review had shared views about the aim of postnatal care including the promotion of maternal health, and the provision of education and advice in relation to women caring for their baby and themselves. The provision of information and support with breastfeeding and parenting skills was raised consistently as one of the main aims of early postnatal care. There was a good deal of congruence in women's and midwives' views in relation to what makes for the most satisfying experience for women – with the relationship and interactions with caregivers raised by the majority of the midwives interviewed. Midwives clearly articulated the barriers associated with providing care in the way that they wished to. These included both organisational issues including understaffing, inadequate staff–patient ratios, required checklists and documentation, interruptions to women's rest by visitors and the diversity of women's needs, including increasing number of women recovering from Caesarean section and the identification and support of women with a range of complex psychosocial issues. There was a strong sense that hospital-based postnatal care is considered a low priority compared with the other episodes of care (Rayner *et al.* 2008).

Making a difference: enhancing early postnatal care

The literature reviewed in this chapter indicates that the way care is structured, the approach to individualised care, the promotion of continuity of care, and the emphasis on quality interactions with caregivers, impact on women' views and experiences of care. Women value

- being treated as individuals;
- continuity of care and caregiver;
- being cared for by caregivers who are sensitive, respectful and understanding;
- care that is provided in a timely and non-rushed manner;
- caregivers who really listen to women and their concerns;
- that their concerns about their own health or that of their baby's health and progress are acknowledged and taken seriously;
- that care and advice is consistent;
- support in relation to the transition from hospital to home.

The challenge is to reorganise early postnatal care to act on these findings. What does it take to shift care from that which is structured and organised to suit the health-care facility or the care provider to one that is women-centred and individualised to meet the needs of each woman?

The 2006 UK national survey of women's experience of maternity care concludes that to move forward on improving care, that health professionals and policymakers should consider women's responses to the survey and the importance of the following:

- *Listening to women as an integral part of care*
- *Remembering and learning from what women say they take away with them*
- *Treating women as individuals with kindness and respect*
- *Continuing to ask women about their views and listening to what they have to say about their care, locally and nationally*

(Redshaw *et al.* 2007)

Health policy in the United Kingdom has highlighted the need to engage health users, making the user perspective central to service design, delivery and evaluation (NICE 2006; Redshaw *et al.* 2007; United Kingdom Department of Health 2007). Women have played a critical role in the evaluation of maternity care. The challenge now is to reorientate postnatal care, taking into account women's views and experiences, and to provide genuine opportunities to engage women and their families in the design and implementation of reform to this vitally important episode of health care.

Conclusion

A key message from this chapter is that both women and midwives place value on care that is tailored to the needs of each individual. Thus postnatal care should be delivered with individualised care as the primary aim, with the full involvement and participation of women. While this seems a relatively straightforward aim, it is clear that numerous barriers impact on the provision of woman-centred postnatal care.

Recognition of the postnatal period as a critically important time for women and their social, physical and emotional health is the first step to improving care. Taking into account the views of women and providers is crucial in the development of reforms to reorientate postnatal care.

Key implications for midwifery practice

- postnatal practitioners need to be highly skilled in assessing and providing support to women with physical, emotional and social health issues following birth.
- postnatal care should be tailored to the needs of each individual woman, with the full participation of women in defining those needs and planning care.
- In considering approaches to reorientating postnatal care, it is critical that the views and experiences of women are taken into account.

References

Bick D (2004) Content and organisation of postnatal care. In: Henderson C, Macdonald S (eds). *Mayes' Midwifery: A Textbook for Midwives*. London: Churchill Livingstone.

Billingham K, Hall D (1998) Turbulent future for school nursing and health visiting. *British Medical Journal* 316: 406–407.

Biro MA, Waldenström U, Brown S, Pannifex JH (2003) Satisfaction with Team Midwifery Care for low- and high-risk women: a randomised controlled trial. *Birth* 30: 1–10.

Boulvain M, Perneger T, Othenin-Girard V, *et al.* (2004) Home-based versus hospital-based postnatal care: a randomised trial. *British Journal of Obstetrics and Gynaecology* 111: 807–813.

Bramadat I, Driedger M (1993) Satisfaction with childbirth: theories and methods of measurement. *Birth* 20 (1): 22–29.

Brooten D, Roncolli M, Finkler S, *et al.* (1994) A randomized trial of early hospital discharge and home follow-up of women having caesarean birth. *Obstetrics and Gynecology* 84 (5): 832–839.

Brown S, Bruinsma F, Darcy M, *et al.* (2004a) Early discharge: no evidence of adverse outcomes in three consecutive population-based Australian surveys of recent mothers. *Paediatric and Perinatal Epidemiology* 18: 202–213.

Brown S, Small R, Faber B, *et al.* (2004b) Early postnatal discharge from hospital for healthy mothers and term infants (Cochrane Review). *The Cochrane Library* 1.

Brown S, Lumley J (1997) The 1993 Survey of Recent Mothers: issues in design, analysis and influencing policy. *International Journal for Quality in Health Care* 9: 265–277.

Brown S, Lumley J (1998) Changing childbirth: lessons from an Australian survey of 1336 women. *British Journal of Obstetrics and Gynaecology* 105: 143–155.

Brown S, Small R, Argus B, *et al.* (2009) Early postnatal discharge from hospital for healthy mothers and term infants (Cochrane Review). *Cochrane Database of Systematic Reviews* 2.

Brown SJ, Darcy M-A, Bruinsma FJ (2005) Women's views and experiences of postnatal hospital care in the Victorian Survey of Recent Mothers 2000. *Midwifery* 21: 109–126.

Bruinsma F, Brown S, Darcy M (2003) Having a baby in Victoria 1989–2000: women's views of public and private models of care. *Australian and New Zealand Journal of Public Health* 27: 20–26.

Cape K (1999) Birth in a new country. In: Rice P (eds). *Asian Mothers, Western Birth*. Melbourne: Ausmed Publications.

Carr-Hill RA (1992) The measurement of patient satisfaction. *Journal of Public Health Medicine* 14 (3): 236–249.

Carty E, Bradley C (1990) A randomized, controlled evaluation of early postpartum hospital discharge. *Birth* 17 (4): 199–204.

Catrell R, Lavender T, Wallymahmead A, *et al.* (2005) Postnatal care: what matters to midwives. *British Journal of Midwifery* 13 (4): 206–213.

Christiaens W, Bracke P (2007) Place of birth and satisfaction with childbirth in Belgium and the Netherlands. *Midwifery*. doi: 1016/j.midw.2007.02.001.

Crow R, Gage H, Hampson S, *et al.* (2002) The measurement of satisfaction with healthcare: Implications for practice from a systematic review of the literature. *Health Technology Assessment* 6 (32), pp6.

Darcy M-A, Brown S, Bruinsma F, Lumley J (2001) *Victorian Survey of Recent Mothers 2000 – 2005: Having a Baby in Metropolitan and Rural Victoria.* Melbourne: Centre for the Study of Mothers' and Children's Health, La Trobe University.

Dykes F (2005) A critical ethnography study of encounters between midwives and breast-feeding women in postnatal wards in England. *Midwifery* 21 (3): 241–252.

Escobar G, Braveman P, Ackerson L, *et al.* (2001) A randomized comparison of home visits and hospital-based group follow-up visits after early postpartum discharge. *Pediatrics* 108 (3): 719–727.

Fishman C, Evans R, Jenks E (1988) Warm bodies, cool milk: conflicts in post partum food choice for Indochinese women in California. *Social Science and Medicine* 26 (11): 1125–1132.

Flint C, Poulengeris P, Grant A (1989) The "Know Your Midwife" scheme – a randomised trial of continuity of care by a team of midwives. *Midwifery* 5: 11–16.

Forster D, McLachlan H, Rayner J, *et al.* (2008) The early postnatal period: exploring women's views, expectations and experiences of care using focus groups in Victoria, Australia. *BMC Pregnancy and Childbirth* 8 (27): 1–17.

Forster D, McLachlan H, Yelland J, *et al.* (2005) *A Review of In-hospital Postnatal Care in Victoria. Final Report.* Melbourne: La Trobe University.

Forster D, Rayner J, Yelland J, *et al.* (2007) *A 'Patient Preference' Approach to Individualised, Flexible Postnatal Care: Exploring Women's Views Using Focus Groups.* Melbourne: Mother and Child Health Research, La Trobe University.

Gagnon A, Edgar L, Kramer M, *et al.* (1997) A randomized trial of a program of early postpartum discharge with nurse visitation. *American Journal of Obstetrics and Gynecology* 176: 205–211.

Garcia J (1999) Mothers' views and experiences of care. In: Marsh G, Renfrew M (eds). *Community-based Maternity Care.* Oxford: Oxford University Press.

Garcia J, Renshaw M, Fitzsimons B, Keene J (1998) *First Class Delivery: A National Survey of Women's Views of Maternity Care.* London: Audit Commission Publications.

Green J, Coupland V, Kitzinger J (1988) *Great Expectations: A Prospective Study of Women's Expectations and Experiences of Childbirth.* Cambridge: Child Care and Development Group.

Green JM, Coupland VA, Kitzinger JV (1990) Expectations, experiences, and psychological outcomes of childbirth: a prospective study of 825 women. *Birth* 17 (1): 15–23.

Green J, Renfrew M, Curtis P (2000) Continuity of carer: what matters to women? A review of the evidence. *Midwifery* 16: 186–196.

Harvey S, Brant R, Stainton C (1996) A randomized, controlled trial of nurse-midwife care. *Birth* 23 (3): 128–135.

Hicks C, Spurgeon P, Barwell F (2003) Changing childbirth: a pilot project. *Journal of Advanced Nursing* 42 (6): 617–628.

Homer C, Davis G, Cooke M, Barclay L (2002a) Women's experiences of continuity of midwifery care in a randomised controlled trial in Australia. *Midwifery* 18: 102–112.

Homer C, Sheehan A, Cooke M (2002b) Initial infant feeding decisions and duration of breastfeeding in women from English, Arabic and Chinese-speaking backgrounds in Australia. *Breastfeed Review* 10: 27–32.

Jacoby A, Cartwright A (1990) Finding out about the views and experiences of maternity-service users. In: Garcia J, Kilpatrick R, Richards M (eds). *The Politics of Maternity Care: Services for Childbearing Women in Twentieth Century Britain*. Oxford: Oxford University Press.

Lauver D, Ward S, Heidrich S, *et al.* (2002) Patient-centred interventions. *Research in Nursing and Health* 25 (4): 246–255.

Lazarus E, Phillipson E (1990) A longitudinal study comparing prenatal care of Puerto Rican and white women. *Birth* 17: 6–11.

Locker D, Dunt D (1978) Theoretical and methodological issues in sociological studies of consumer satisfaction with medical care. *Social Science and Medicine* 12: 283–292.

Lumley J (1985) Assessing satisfaction with childbirth. *Birth* 12 (3): 141–145.

MacArthur C, Winter HR, Bick DE, *et al.* (2002) Effects of redesigned community postnatal care on women's health 4 months after birth: a cluster randomised controlled trial. *Lancet* 359: 378–371.

MacArthur C, Winter HR, Bick DE, *et al.* (2003) *Redesigning Postnatal Care; A Randomised Controlled Trial of Protocol Based, Midwifery Led Care Focused on Individual Women's Physical and Psychological Health Needs*. Southampton, England: NHS R and D, NCC HTA.

Marchant S (2003) Physiology and care in the puerperium. In: Fraser D, Cooper M (eds). *Myles Textbook for Midwives*. London: Bailliere Tindall.

McLachlan H, Forster D (2006) Initial breastfeeding attitudes and practices of women born in Turkey, Vietnam and Australia after giving birth in Australia. *International Breastfeeding Journal* 1 (7).

McLachlan H, Forster D, Davey M, *et al.* (2008) COSMOS: comparing standard maternity care with one-to-one midwifery support: a randomised controlled trial. *BMC Pregnancy and Childbirth* 8 (35). doi: 10.1186/1471-2393-8-35.

Murray D, Ryan F, Keane E (2000) Who's holding the baby? Women's experiences of their postnatal care. *Irish Medical Journal* 93 (5): 148–150.

National Institute for Health and Clinical Excellence (2006) *Routine Post-natal Care of Women and their Babies. Clinical Guideline 37*, London, available at: http://www.nice.org.uk/CG037 (accessed 11/10/2007).

Oakley A (1979) *Becoming a Mother*. Oxford: Martin Robertson.

Porter M, Macintyre S (1984) What is, must be best: A research note on conservative or deferential responses to antenatal care provision. *Social Science & Medicine* 19 (11): 1197–1200.

Proctor S (1998) What determines quality in maternity care? Comparing the perceptions of childbearing women and midwives. *Birth* 25 (2): 85–93.

Rayner J-A, Forster D, McLachlan H, *et al.* (2008) A state-wide review of hospital postnatal care in Victoria, Australia: the views and experiences of midwives. *Midwifery* 24: 310–320.

Redshaw M, Rowe R, Hockley C, Brocklehurst P (2007) *Recorded Delivery: A National Survey of Women's Experience of Maternity Care 2006*. Oxford: National Perinatal Epidemiology Unit, University of Oxford.

Rice P (1999) Childbirth and health: cultural beliefs and practices among Cambodian women. In: Rice P (eds). *Asian Mothers, Western Birth*. Melbourne: Ausmed Publications.

Rowley M, Hensley M, Brinsmead M, Wlodarczyk J (1995) Continuity of care by a midwife team versus routine care during pregnancy and birth: a randomised trial. *Medical Journal of Australia* 163: 289–293.

Rudman A, El-Khouri B, Waldenstrom U (2007) Evaluating multi-dimensional aspects of postnatal hospital care. *Midwifery*, 24 (4); 425–441.

Sitzia J, Wood N (1997) Patient satisfaction: a review of issues and concepts. *Social Science and Medicine* 45 (12): 1829–1843.

Small R, Rice P, Yelland J, Lumley J (1999) Mothers in a new country: the role of culture and communication in Vietnamese, Turkish and Filipino women's experiences of giving birth in Australia. *Women and Health* 28: 77–101.

Small R, Yelland J, Lumley J, Rice P (1997) *Mothers in a New Country: Vietnamese, Turkish and Filipino Women's Views of Maternity Care*. Melbourne: Centre for the Study of Mothers' and Children's Health.

Stamp GE, Crowther CA (1994) Women's views of their postnatal care by midwives at an Adelaide Women's Hospital. *Midwifery* 10: 148–156.

Steel O'Connor K, Mowat D, Scott H, *et al.* (2003) A randomised trial of two public health nurse follow-up programs of early obstetrical discharge. *Canadian Journal of Public Health* 94 (2): 98–103.

Sullivan D, Beeman R (1982) Satisfaction with maternity care: a matter of communication and choice. *Medical Care* 20 (3): 321–330.

Tran M, Young L, Phung H, *et al.* (2001) Quality of health services and early post-partum discharge: results from a sample of non-English-speaking women. *Journal of Quality Clinical Practice* 21: 135–143.

Turnbull D, Holmes A, Shields N, *et al.* (1996) Randomised, controlled trial of efficacy of midwife-managed care. *Lancet* 348: 213–218.

United Kingdom Department of Health (2007) *Maternity Matters: Choice, Access and Continuity of Care in a Safe Service*. London: Department of Health.

Waldenström U, Brown S, McLachlan H, *et al.* (2000) Does team midwife care increase satisfaction with antenatal, intrapartum and postnatal care? A randomised controlled trial. *Birth* 27: 156–167.

Waldenstrom U, Lindmark G (1987) Early and late discharge after hospital birth: a comparative study of parental background characteristics. *Scandinavian Journal of Social Medicine* 1987 (15): 159–167.

Waldenstrom U, Rudman A, Hildingsson I (2006) Intrapartum and postpartum care in Sweden: women's opinions and risk factors for not being satisfied. *Acta Obstetricia et Gynecologica Scandinavica* 85: 551–600.

Waldenström U, Turnbull D (1998) A systematic review comparing continuity of midwifery care with standard maternity services. *British Journal of Obstetrics and Gynaecology* 105: 1160–1170.

Wiggins M, Oakley A, Roberts I, *et al.* (2004) The social support and family health study: a randomised controlled trial and economic evaluation of two alternative forms of postnatal support for mothers living in disadvantaged inner-city areas. *Health Technology Assessment* 8: 32.

Woollett A, Dosanjh-Matwala N (1990) Postnatal care: the attitudes and experiences of Asian women in east London. *Midwifery* 90: 178–184.

Yelland J, Krastev A, Brown S (2009) Enhancing early postnatal care: findings from a major reform of maternity care in three Australian hospitals. *Midwifery* 25: 392–402.

Yelland J, Small R, Lumley J, *et al.* (1998) Support, sensitivity, satisfaction: Filipino, Turkish and Vietnamese women's experiences of postnatal hospital stay. *Midwifery* 14: 144–154.

Chapter 4
Transition into Parenthood: Ideology and Reality

Kathryn Gutteridge

Introduction – becoming a mother

Becoming a mother is perhaps the most challenging life transition that a woman will ever make. Adolescence with all its mood adjustments and physical changes does little to prepare for the childbirth crisis and separation of a woman and her body during pregnancy. How does it happen? The body appears to surge ahead with its physiological demands but how does the mind run alongside this phenomenon? This mystery is relatively undiscovered; it is unique and exclusive from one woman to another.

In this chapter, we attempt to understand the psychological changes women go through in becoming a mother. This incorporates early pregnancy, experiences that aid the process and the problems that bearing a child in the twenty-first century creates. In examining the pregnancy, we explore the preparation for birth and how that experience influences mothering, including important aspects such as birth and infant feeding. We examine maternal and infant attachment processes, what it means and where there are problems, how this might affect the future relationship of mother and child. In conclusion, we examine the role of fatherhood and how this relationship fits within a parenting framework. Underpinning this transition is the role of the midwife, this unique and dynamic relationship, which is integral to women's adjustment to motherhood.

From me to mother – exploring what this means

In discovering her pregnancy a woman will make a huge dynamic shift in thinking, she may experience shock, fear, uncertainty and perhaps joy. All of these emotions flood through the mind and may create a state of intense fear even for a short time; this does not mean that she does not want her baby but she may experience a brief period of acute panic.

Pregnancy and motherhood is a rite of passage, a necessary part of human life ensuring genetic certainty for future generations. This state is challenged today by complex psychosocial factors. However, Raphael-Leff (2001) describes this essential human experience as seeking to fulfil a series of individual quests:

- Genetic immortality
- Becoming 'adult'

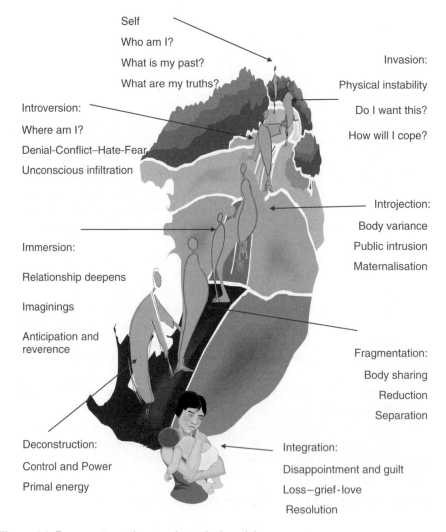

Figure 4.1 From me to mother – a theoretical model.

- Emulating the parent(s)
- Reciprocating parental care
- Sharing a 'second chance'
- Love object
- Cultural transmission

Motherhood brings with it expectations and dreams, it is a social proclamation of female maturity and an opportunity to pass on our knowledge, skills and stories of womanly experiences.

Already in this short span of time, women are beginning an attachment process to their infant, which at this early stage in pregnancy, is often described as her ideal baby. She has a relationship with her fetus that is unique and exclusive; this is not to say that the woman loves her baby at this stage but that she is developing a sense of coherence and deep understanding with her child.

The journey of pregnancy may be over but another has begun with constant demands from her infant. Fractured relationships, with both self and others need time to realign and move into a deeper understanding of life. This is woman and motherhood, it is not separate to life before; it is part of it. Pregnancy and childbirth is a complex state; it is a fusion of primal experiences and beginning new attachments for both mother and infant.

Figure 4.1 shows this dynamic journey describing the emotional states.

Modernity and motherhood

Influences that determine when a woman will become pregnant have changed in modern society. Today young women can defer pregnancy and control their fertility in ways that our grandmothers had little choice over. Becoming a mother at the turn of the twentieth century brought real and significant risk of mortality, whereas loss in modern society is perceived in much less of a physical sense and more of a materialistic event.

Fatherhood is a social construct, which is bequeathed, whereas motherhood is physically experienced and witnessed by society, there is no doubt that a woman is inextricably bound to her developing fetus in a way that fathers never could be. This fact may explain some of the patriarchal constructs created to control fertility, childbirth and womanhood (Chodorow 1978). Feminists have long explored and challenged the role of men within fertility and questioned their interference; women are by their nature able to procreate and suckle their babies and therefore perceived to be much closer to nature. This gives women a fixed certainty with their infants, an interconnectedness that is private and excludes the male.

Mother, fetus and infant attachments are described by Kagan (1978) as 'an intense emotional relationship that is specific to the two'. It is important to understand this journey through childbirth and the changes within the female body and psyche, which cement the woman to her infant.

Pregnancy – a female condition?

Raphael-Leff (2001) disputes the use of the term 'condition' – she describes it as a 'process'. This is an important construct in the Western hemisphere, as we exist within a culture that is overly reliant upon technology and medical structures, the influences within pregnancy are significant.

Historically, pregnancy was almost uniquely within the world of women, with the confirmation of pregnancy reliant upon the woman recognising changes within her body. She would have discussed these with her family or peers and their influences would have been evident through pregnancy until the birth of her infant (Kitzinger 2005). In our highly socialised maternity culture, the discovery of pregnancy is commonly handed to others; this may be a chemist, midwife, doctor, or even a TV screen in the case of sonography. This process has distanced women from their bodies with reliance upon others rather than trusting her own instincts.

The majority of knowledge shared with women today is mainly technological and media-driven, creating a distance between feminine cultures and the history of mothering experiences. This is demonstrated in Table 4.1.

All of these factors both in utero and after birth influence maternal/infant attachment. The power of modern maternity services is vast; the concept of insecure attachments, fostering dependencies upon technology or professional input should not be underestimated.

Contrasting opinions in society

Although we have considered pregnancy through this techno-cultural lens it is perhaps worth examining a feminist's perspective in the concept of attachment and motherhood.

When a woman announces her pregnancy to the world, she is often congratulated and treated with respect, even if the pregnancy is invisible to the onlooker. It is a declaration of womanhood; however, the flipside of the coin may be that the more visibly pregnant she appears the less

Table 4.1 An example of control issues within midwifery and childbirth.

Gestation	Technological/ service input	Experiential impact	Locus of control
Pre-pregnant	May be taking contraceptives	Decision not to be pregnant	With woman
Pre-conceptional	Folic acid, diet, smoking cessation, alcohol reduction Ovulation predictors	Decision to try to be pregnant	With woman
Conception	Pregnancy kit	'Blue Line' joy, fear, anticipation, excitement	With woman
5–8 weeks	GP confirms pregnancy midwife, booking history, focus on risk factors, labelling	Seeks confirmation and reassurance	With service
8–12 weeks	Screening information, ultrasound scan	Visual confirmation, dissociates from internal knowledge of own body	With service
12–16 weeks	Screening tests, ultrasound scans. Chemical selection of fetal normality	Fear, anxiety needing reassurance from professionals, dependent upon test results	With service
20 weeks	Detailed anomaly scan	Fear, anxiety, wants to know sex, see fetus on screen, dependent upon sonographer	With service
24 weeks onwards	Regular antenatal visits	Abandoned, seeks reassurance, needs to be told fetus is growing and normal	With service
Birth preparation	Parenting classes, active birth Maternity tours	Near to birth, fear, apprehension, excitement, confusion	With service
Onset of labour	Call midwife, go into hospital Examined for confirmation of labour	Unsure, afraid, in pain, excited, tearful, body is responding to labour	With service
Birth	Menu of pain relief, equipment monitors fetus and mother, augment labour, episiotomy, forceps, ventouse, caesarean section, active management	Sensory perception heightened, coping, afraid, alone, distress, relief, fear of death	With service
Post-birth	Home, midwife visits, health visitor, family	Support needed, body hurting, baby demanding, tired, unsure, seeks reassurance	With baby

tolerant society becomes; where once the woman had her own invisible private space, she now becomes the property of society (Forna 1998).

Examples of this are as follows:

- Unrequested advice from strangers
- Suggestions of what is safe to eat or drink
- When to rest and work

These illustrations lead to a sense that life is controlled by others. The media have a role in the guarding of pregnancy with advertising a powerful tool and one might even describe this as the 'pregnancy police'. Forna (1998) describes pregnancy as being directed away from the mother with all of the attention shifted entirely to the fetus. She further suggests that newspapers' consistency in focusing upon the monitoring of the rights of the fetus denies the role of the mother with powerful headlines such as 'a mother's diet during pregnancy may condemn her child to heart disease decades later'.

A powerful representation of motherhood is the Madonna and Child image; serene smile, body well-covered and contented infant. However, the feminist camp raises powerful challenges; over the last decade the 'A' list celebrity has made pregnancy and childbirth their domain, challenging stereotypes of the past. It is quite normal today to see naked pregnant celebrities engaging in photo shoots, celebrating their pregnancies. These influences are powerful, whereas women of the 1950s might have worn maternity smocks concealing their gravid status, it is commonplace today for young pregnant women to bare their bellies to the world emulating the pregnant celebrity role models.

With that said, there are still pregnancy behaviours that cause public distaste despite celebrating the beauty of the pregnant body. The non-compliant smoking teenage mother, for instance, is an image that raises debate. Secrecy and silence become an everyday part of childbearing with society controlling the behaviours and meting punishment when a woman does not appear to subscribe to putting her unborn child's needs first.

Mothering and the mother

How do we know how to behave and model ourselves when we start the journey of motherhood? Influences come from every aspect of the globe, media, magazines, health professionals, Internet and perhaps most of all from our friends and family. There is none so influential as our parents but particularly the relationship we have with our mothers. Women aspire to be the 'good enough mother', which Winnicott (1957) describes as a capacity for patience, devotion and self-sacrifice and places the future of the child solely in the hands of the mother.

This unique relationship is the template by which our experiences of parenthood are based; we will choose to parent in a way we were raised or conversely reverse those experiences which we found deficient as a child. Our attachment to our parents is complicated, often tempered with love, loyalty, hate and disappointment. Forna (1998) writes, 'mothers have the capacity to disappoint us, anger us, frustrate us and burden us in a way no one else can', in fact, today many individuals seek therapy and the basis of their psychoanalysis is a dysfunctional relationship with their own mother.

In the initial stages of pregnancy, memories of early experiences are evocative with reprocessing of old events played out with ourselves as the mother. Women are inclined to place themselves in the Madonna role, the idealistic mother who is content, capable, sacrificial and wholesome. Unspoken promises made to her fetus for a future life that is free of harm, she will be her child's guardian.

For some pregnant mothers, the absence of any real physical contact with their mothers in their formative years can present a challenge. Motherhood is the most natural physical experience and the emotional responses to her infant may be overwhelming. If the woman's own needs in childhood were ignored, then the ability to respond empathically to her own infant may be impaired. This experience is supported by Sigmund Freud's exploration of the mother/infant relationship, which he explains, 'the reason why the infant in arms wants to perceive the presence of its mother is because it already knows by experience that she satisfies all its needs without delay' (Freud 1926).

Freud (1940a,b) based most of his original theories and psychoanalytical practice upon adult relationship with mothers. His work was the framework for all twentieth-century analysts and today modern psychotherapy is deeply rooted in his philosophical theories. He stated the significance of this relationship and particularly the function of breastfeeding within the maternal role. He described the mother as 'unique, without parallel (and) established unilaterally for a whole lifetime as the first and strongest love-object ... the prototype of all later love reactions' (Freud 1926). Others were to follow in the exploration of this very complex relationship.

Melanie Klein, fundamentally a great supporter of Freud, continued to investigate the relationship between mother and daughter. She herself was an unwanted child and received little affection from her parents, later seeking psychoanalysis she became academically involved within this field and wrote at length about the mother/infant affiliation (Klein 1998). The relationship with the infant and the mother's breast is famously dysfunctional according to Klein; 'the power of love – is there in the baby as well as the destructive impulses, and finds its first fundamental expression in the baby's attachment to his mother's breast, which develops into love for her as a person' (Klein 1998).

Complex though this is, in its simplicity motherhood is incredibly powerful and influential. Infant behaviours are mediated by the presence of mothering, responding to basic human needs such as warmth, food and touch. Albert Maslow's (1943) humanist theory describes these basic human states as 'deficiency needs'; these have to be met in order to function, the provision of food outstrips that of love. However, if food is regularly supplied but there is no human attention to love and emotional stimulation, there is a problem.

> The pregnant woman is beginning to provide her unborn infant with its basic needs, she is eating for two, resting when advised and taking advantage of health services that will guide her and protect the well-being of baby. She may be unaware of her nurturing at this point but she is sending strong messages to her fetus that she cares and that she will provide all it needs.
>
> Maslow's (1943) Hierarchy of Needs

Origins of attachment in pregnancy

> Antenatal care has become a rigorous screening event with evidence-based interventions that bind women to the service. The reduction of infant and maternal mortality has largely been ascribed to the success of antenatal screening and risk assessment-based care. It is no wonder that women are persuaded by antenatal care; we provide them with pictures of their unborn baby, which may even be put to music or screening tests that can predict a *'perfect baby'*. If women decide they do not want screening or some aspect of care we name them as 'deviants' or non-compliant; naming and shaming them
>
> (Wolf 2001)

There is no doubt that maternal/infant attachment begins its journey early in pregnancy. The physical changes of pregnancy are influenced by the hormonal and biochemical ebb and flow, which supports not only the changing body but also the psychological adjustments. Raphael-Leff (2001) theorises that the physical symptoms of pregnancy generate psychological interpretations by women such as resenting the fetus for making her nauseous or sick. She further describes pregnancy-related psychological experiences in three maturational phases as follows:

1. Phase one – 'the emphasis is on the pregnancy; psychological manifestations are emotional disequilibrium, preoccupations with body image, food, telling others'.
2. Phase two – 'emphasis shifts from the pregnancy to the fetus, now experienced as separate. She may be excited and fascinated by the movements and her visible body changes; she pats and soothes her fundus'.

3. Phase three – 'the woman starts to visualise the baby existing outside of her body and she becomes preoccupied with the emotional and physical preparation for birth. The baby becomes real and shifts from an imaginary or fantasy infant. Primitive bodily anxieties emerge, which, if unresolved, may affect labour'.

A sense of knowingness emerges throughout pregnancy, a relationship that mother and fetus develop. This rapport is incremental as both observe each other's pattern of activity and develop an appreciation of each other's habits. It is well known that the fetus responds in utero to loud stimuli such as music and vibrations, but now we also understand the impact of maternal stressors and catecholamine biochemical surges upon fetal activity (Field *et al.* 2006). There is significant evidence to show that persistent levels of stress hormones have a long-term impact upon fetal outcomes and consequently affect their childhood development (Gerhardt 2004).

Smoking in pregnancy is a good example – researchers have demonstrated that the fetus becomes agitated when a mother inhales a cigarette; the theory is based upon the fact that during a smoking episode placental oxygen level diminishes and therefore heightens fetal distress (Lieberman *et al.* 1992).

In response to stress chemicals, the fetus increases its movements; however, if maternal anxiety continues, there is an expectation that there will be an increased prevalence of premature birth and that the fetus will suffer intrauterine growth retardation, and even mimic the mother's prenatal biochemical/physiological profile including elevated cortisol, lower levels of dopamine and serotonin (Field *et al.* 2006).

Maternal anxiety to some degree is normal; its roots are found in a desire to be the 'good mother'; however, the nature of modern childbearing could mean that women are exposed to significant stressors above that, which is considered normal. The 'pregnancy police' place a huge responsibility upon women whose every action is scrutinised and observed; any deviations are publicly confirmed (Forna 1998). This factor cannot help but interfere with the way a woman might perceive her pregnancy and fetus, ultimately determining the relationship she might have with her child.

Imaginings, fantasies and 'dream baby'

In early pregnancy, women dream about their 'baby to be'; this is based upon idealisations of their baby and negative fears. The pregnant sub-consciousness is actively magnified; Wolf (2001) describes her dreams containing 'vivid characters and wilder scenes' than ever dreamed in her non-pregnant life. She suggests that dreams prepare women for motherhood and this is confirmed by other researchers (Sered & Abramovitch 1992).

There appears to be an increasing urgency in dreams as a pregnancy progresses with reports of losing the baby when out walking or that the baby might be born with bizarre features (Sered & Abramovitch 1992).

The phenomenon of vivid dreams in pregnancy is reportedly due to the changing pattern of sleep and increased level of progesterone and oestrogen. These two pregnancy-rich hormones influence rapid eye movement (REM) which is associated with dream patterns. An individual sleeps in cycles of non-rapid eye movement (NREM) and REM and would, usually within 8 hours of sleep, experience 4–5 cycles of REM, up to approximately 20% of sleep time.

Sleep is influenced during pregnancy by discomfort from the gravid uterus, bladder frequency and generalised sleep change in readiness for early motherhood. However, the effect of pregnancy hormones are reported to result in elongated phases of REM and may therefore help to explain the enhanced quality and recall of dreams experienced during pregnancy. This can be disturbing for some women and they often need reassurance about the changes in their dream pattern and content.

Whether dreams are comforting or disturbing Raphael-Leff (2001) considers this aspect of motherhood a natural feature of maternal/infant attachment. Raphael-Leff theorises that this concept splits into three distinct components 'positive prenatal, neutral and negative' attachment experiences.

- Positive prenatal attachment – is dependent on how much the pregnant woman invests in herself and how her capacity for trust is rooted in a positive outcome. This means she will 'fall in love' with her fetus and her fantasy of the child is fulfilled by becoming her dream baby.
- Neutral attachment – this is where the pregnant woman suspends her fantasies just in case the reality does not measure up. Her dreams may reflect her fears; she might fantasise the birth ending not with a baby but just with a blood clot or piece of tissue. She may be protecting herself or even her other children, she could have experienced some other negative pregnancy outcomes.
- Negative attachment – this is explained as being constantly preoccupied with waking and sleeping negative dreams. She might lack confidence in her body and ability to have babies. She might describe her fetus in conflict with her own bodily needs. She is unconvinced of her worth as a mother to be and can experience a pregnancy burdened with competing anxieties, dreams and fears, even desiring to end the life of her fetus.

While dreams of the fetus are common, some women have vivid thoughts about their placenta. Physiologically the placenta is a critical aspect of pregnancy; it nourishes, protects and breathes life into the fetus. Interestingly, some women focus on nurturing their placenta as well as their fetus. They may see the food they eat ingested first by their placenta and then processed for their infant; this may be reinforced by antenatal advice about what to eat for a healthy pregnancy outcome. Indeed some women may describe their fetus disliking some foods that they eat; for instance, 'my baby gets hiccoughs when I eat oranges'. This might seem an irrational explanation; however, the mother is forming her own understanding and attachment to her unborn child's tastes and behaviours.

Many women do not understand the detailed functioning of the placenta but will have imaginings of this organ and how it serves the fetus. Hunger cravings easily explained are more likely to be described by pregnant women as a need to feed their developing fetus: 'eating for two'. Food becomes a focus with waves of nausea and desperate hunger swings. She is forming a strong unconscious relationship with her baby and the magical belief that she is nourishing her infant.

Dreams, fantasies and imaginings are a reality of pregnancy and motherhood attachment processes; it is the beginning of a complicated affiliation between mother and fetus.

Fetal movements – in utero communication and listening to mother

The first time a fetus moves is a significant event in pregnancy awaited with interest by mother, family and professional. Women often describe fetal movements as 'butterflies or gurgling'; however, they are soon distinguishable as those of the baby. During antenatal appointments, enquiries about the presence of fetal movements are routine and women are encouraged to monitor them daily. Once fetal movements are felt, the emphasis shifts from the pregnancy to the reality of a developing baby. The woman may have internal conversations with her fetus; she may be observed stroking and caressing her growing uterus and even talking to her baby. Although physically unable to feel the baby's movements, the father is not totally excluded; he might feel and even witness the baby kicking.

The pattern of fetal movements are subconsciously noted and regulated by the woman's day-to-day activities; she soon becomes accustomed to the behaviour of her growing baby. The comfort derived from this behaviour is significant; it forms part of the maturing relationship and attachment between mother and child.

There are suggestions that the concept of maternal/fetal attachment during ultrasound investigation is enhanced by visualisation; however,

Baillie *et al.* (1996) dispute this. Researchers found there was little substantiation to support ultrasonography for maternal/fetal bonding, in fact, in some aspects of research it had an opposing view. This is explained by the fact that women experiencing pregnancy problems and exposed to more frequent scans are more often than not increasingly anxious, even worried and depressed (Clement *et al.* 1998). It appears that the presence of regular movements and an internal knowledge that the fetus responds to the mother's voice is much more influential (De Casper & Fifer 1980; Benassi *et al.* 2004). The accessibility of fetal stethoscopes, which can be purchased from high street stores, has opened up another debate. The ability to auscultate the fetal heart in the intimacy of a couple's own home is increasing, this practice means that getting to know their baby is within their own grasp and less dependent on a midwife. The danger here is that knowledge is limited and anxiety may be heightened when the woman is unable to find the fetal heart.

While fetal movements may provide pregnant women with reassurance and a sense of comfort, there are those women for whom the whole concept of a growing fetus inside their womb will fill them with disgust. With a history of rape, sexual assault or incest the active fetus will challenge the way a woman views herself. Women who have become pregnant because of rape may experience psychological trauma when the fetus moves, a constant reminder of the experience.

Sexual abuse, whether in adulthood or during childhood, has a long-lasting impact upon the development of adult self-esteem. Self-worth and confidence is affected and a range of psychological issues emerge at different times in a survivor's life. Becoming pregnant with an unwanted child is a huge burden for a woman to bear but nonetheless a choice many women will face and endure. The presence of a growing and moving fetus raises many physical and psychological dilemmas.

Fetal movements are particularly difficult for some survivors, Rose (1992) describes the movements of her baby which was conceived through incestuous rape as 'like an alien growing inside me and invading my body, each time it moved I felt physically sick and dirty'.

It is evident that some women find little comfort in both the changing body image and physicality of their pregnancies; it is best to avoid assumptions in relation to how women respond to their fetuses. Dissociating from fetal movements is more common than known and some women adopt this practice in order to cope with private feelings of disgust.

There is a wide spectrum of emotion that pregnant women experience from their fetal movements; ranging from pleasure in looking inside of the womb (ultrasound scan) to horror when the baby kicks. Some women have a real sense of purpose and knowingness about their growing baby; however, for others it presents a real psychodynamic challenge.

Birth – a crisis

Anticipating the birth of a child is a step into the unknown; education and preparation may help in terms of labour but that does not **prepare** for the psychological leap women make. The thought of labour and its associated pain may cause fear, particularly if it is the first birth where women may wonder as to how they will cope.

Birth is such a transforming experience that women recall memories of the event for many years, often into their old age. Simkin (1991) in her enlightening work with women of all ages found that they had clear and concise recall of their birth experiences even remembering what had been said by whom. This, in part, is due to the intense production of oxytocin during labour, which enhances the amygdyla, a part of the limbic system, which stores memories for later recall. This psychodynamic effect is powerful in the establishment of healthy attachments, particularly if the memories are good.

Women who are confident and relaxed when in labour will meet their new infant in a way that supports this healthy relationship. There is a great deal of agreement about the value of support during labour; this is demonstrated when observing women encouraged to let go of their inhibitions and follow the instinctual nature of labour. When anxious and fearful, she is more likely to be working against her body and ultimately transfer her feelings to her baby in utero. Although women expect labour to be painful, the ability to cope with it and overcome is dependent upon the quality of caregiver support and the environment in which birth takes place.

Michel Odent has long studied birth and the way it manifests when natural environments dominate. He based much of his original theory on mammals who seek dark, warm and secluded spaces to give birth to their young. He suggests that when these variables are present hormones natural to labour are at their peak and will facilitate a normal outcome. In Odent's (1991) observations into labouring mammals, he noted that if regional anaesthesia was used during the labour process, the impact on attachment with their young was significant, they failed to care as well for their offspring.

Women have to overcome many factors in achieving the best circumstances for birth to take place: bright lights, poor communication and lack of support, which make the task harder. Nature has provided women with a complex neurophysical process initiated only during labour; the neocortex is rested so that primitive brain structures can easily release the necessary labour hormones. The effect of this biochemical change enables women to dissociate from their surroundings and follow primitive urges necessary for birth. Inhibitions of daily life are abandoned; it is common for women to find themselves in the most unexpected, often primitive postures. The environment that facilitates the best birth outcomes will also enable the woman in the relationship with her new baby.

The final throes of labour are testament to the courage of women, the power of the uterus and the determination of the fetus to be born. Odent (1978) refers to the 'fetus ejection reflex' or transitional stage of labour in which the woman lapses into a transitory state of fear and irrational behaviour. According to Odent, one of the factors, which may interfere with this process is the environment and unwanted communication. Women will often adopt an upright position at this point; there is a huge surge in hormone levels, particularly oxytocin and adrenaline, as she experiences uncontrollable urges to push her baby out. The woman is very close to her baby at this point, she is visualising the welcome she is about to make to her baby.

The trend for father support during labour is a distraction for labouring women, Odent (1978) states; 'birth is traditionally an all-female event' and that social pressures now force fathers to be present. Niven (1992) researched women's views on partner support during labour and discovered a small number of women did find it unhelpful to have their partners with them. However, the majority of women in the study said that their pain and anxiety was lower if their partner (male or female) was present. This information is important when caring for labouring women and their partners particularly when bringing a family together for the first time.

Once the baby is emerging, the woman may feel a reluctance to thrust her baby for the final few pushes, a normal sense of fear and panic. Once the presenting part is clear of the perineum the woman is wide awake and in the last few seconds pushes her baby into the world. The midwife placing her baby upon her chest is starting the very process of physical attachment between mother and infant, it is a critical aspect of uniting the two. This is where the physical meeting of dreams are realised, sometimes with disappointment but more often than not with relief at a safe birth outcome. This process in enhanced where the mother is able to 'catch' her own baby as is common with the practice of waterbirths; she is the first person to touch her baby and makes that immediate connection.

Attachment and bonding – theory and reality

The first few seconds after the birth between mother and infant are fascinating; it is a time of mutual urgency. The mother has a need to know that her baby is safe and physically well, the baby is making tremendous adaptations to life. If the infant is next to its mother's skin, the critical aspects of attachment are initiated.

Ethologist Lorenz (1935) first introduced attachment as a theory; in his studies of non-humans, he found that the subject made a strong attachment to the first object seen after birth. While the attachment object is usually the mother, it may not always be the case as precocial species are able to form attachments without feeding; Lorenz called this process *imprinting*. Bornstein (1989) further supports this theory of attachment in adding a dimension of a 'critical period' in which this experience takes place, this is vital for the normal neurological development of the infant.

Moving Lorenz's theory forward, John Bowlby studied and applied the experience of human attachment based on 'imprinting' into a more useful framework. Bowlby (1969) stated that because human infants are born helpless they are genetically programmed to behave towards their mothers in ways that ensure their survival. He went further to suggest that mothers are also programmed to respond to the helplessness of their baby and there is a critical period when this should occur to form the basis of their attachment. Once this attachment is formed, mother and infant are regulated by each other, involving how far a mother can tolerate being away from her child and how fearful the child will be in its mother's absence. Bowlby (1951) states; 'mother love in infancy is as important for mental health as are vitamins and proteins for physical health'.

Klaus and Kennell (1976) add further weight to the work of Bowlby in discussing the 'maternal sensitive' period. This research was instrumental in hospital practices of allowing mothers to 'room in' with their infants, whereby previously babies were all cared for in a nursery. However, subsequent research has doubted the existence of a critical time for this sensitive period and found no long-term effects of early separation (Rutter 1981). This is contested in later studies of maternal infant separation, for instance, babies requiring care in neonatal units, where mothers have limited access where touch, cuddling and feeding is restricted. Not only is this thought to affect the infant but this also might significantly influence the mother's physical and mental well-being (Affleck & Tennen 1991).

The experience of women giving birth in the theatre by caesarean section is another example where attachment, bonding and interaction is interrupted. Today, most couples are together in the theatre for the birth unless there is a need to perform an emergency caesarean under general anaesthetic. The use of sterile procedures, a screen placed at the level of the mother's breasts and resuscitaires placed out of sight is commonplace. What these practices are likely to create is a separation of the experience of birth from the mother. It is common for others to see the baby before the mother, pass the baby to the partner before the mother and wrap the baby and therefore skin-to-skin contact has to wait. Some women have even experienced doubt about the baby belonging to them, particularly if resuscitation has occurred and the baby taken to a neonatal unit. It is vital that we approach birth even in situations of emergency that aspire to unite mother and infant in their attachment to each other.

Ainsworth *et al.* (1978) believe that attachment is 'an essential part of the ground plan of the human species for an infant to become attached to a mother figure'; however, she states that this does not have to be a biological mother. Ainsworth studied attachment alongside Bowlby and is perhaps most famous for the 'strange situation' observation. This study used close observation of a mother and her 1-year-old infant, the mother and baby are put through a series of actions, and at one point the mother leaves the infant alone in the room. She defined the following:

- Securely attached infants – who cry or protest when mothers leave the room and greet her happily when returning.
- Avoidant infants – who rarely cry when the mother leaves and avoid her on return to the room.
- Ambivalent or resistant infants – who are anxious before the mother leaves the room and upset when she leaves; however, are ambivalent when she returns by seeking contact with her but at the same time hitting out.

Attachment is established from a working model, this is what an infant can expect of its mother, the routines she develops and the periods of close contact. Secure attachment is influenced by the mother through affectionate and responsive behaviour to her infant, positive interaction is thought to be more significant than the amount of time a mother spends with her infant. Ainsworth found that this sensitivity was by far the most important aspect of secure attachment; she observed that these mothers hold their babies closer to them and feed them on the baby's cue rather than time related.

However important the infant considers its mother, it is evident that the baby is able to develop multiple significant attachments necessary for its survival and development. Bowlby's theory on monotropy (where infants develop a strong innate tendency to become attached and respond only to its mother) has been criticised and disputed, Schaffer and Emerson (1964) found that multiple attachments are possible and while not necessarily as strong as with the mother, nonetheless, are just as important. Bowlby was dismissive of the father role and considered it unimportant in the child's development. Lamb (1978), however, found that fathering was as effective as mothering and is negligible in the way a child develops attachments to constant caregivers.

Many factors are influential in the attachment process none less so than the mother's social support systems. The reason a woman decides to have her baby, her past life experiences, emotional states, and relationship with the baby's father – are important factors influencing the relationship she develops with her baby.

Hello baby – welcome to my world

When a mother meets her baby for the first time there is a whole raft of emotion ranging from relief that labour is over to excitement as her baby is placed in her arms. There are those women who are indifferent to their infants; however, emotions that are more positive emerge within days as caretaking and feeding establishes. Particularly in modern birthing units outside of the home, a mother's emotions are influenced by other factors such as harsh lighting, medications and unfamiliar noise. All of these issues serve to interfere with the way mothers and babies greet each other.

Raphael-Leff (2001) describes mothers following a predictable pattern and order when first greeting their babies; this starts with tactile exploration of the following:

- Hands
- Feet
- Trying to get the baby to open its eyes
- Stroking of face and lips
- Identifying similar features with other family members

The initial alertness of the baby in the first 45 minutes of life is followed by a sleepy state sometimes lasting for days only waking for food. It is during those first few minutes that maternal infant connections are firmly established; however, for some women this time can be confusing. Becoming a mother and indeed parent is not an immediate transition but is a state of organic development.

One of the most important aspects of the mother–infant relationship is that of naming the child. This serves to connect the two but is also a significant factor in the baby developing its own sense of self-identity. The name of the baby may have been already decided and many months of discussion taking place between the parents and family. This process separates the baby from its parents and gives it legal status, although once part of each other, now they are connected only through their pregnancy history.

Introducing a new baby to its family and siblings is an important event within family life. There are important traditions that are observed within some cultures that are practised to welcome the baby to the family. It is important that healthcare professionals are able to embrace these practices within hospital and birthing environments.

Gender differences

There is evidence in Western cultures that parents immediately react to the gender of their babies and indeed a socialisation process commences soon after birth. Raphael-Leff (2001) observed new mothers' reactions to their babies; this depends upon her own experiences of childhood and parenting. She further suggests that if the mother has a female child she will be constrained and influenced by her feelings about her own mother and similarly if giving birth to a male her relationship with her father.

Some cultural aspects of gender influence the welcome the child receives within its new family. If the parents place a great deal of emphasis on a particular sex, then this will be a persuasive factor in the way they nurture and condition their child. Gender socialisation may start as early as infancy with parents using stereotypical language such as 'he's a big boy or she's a little girl'.

Traditionally, in Western cultures, boys are dressed in blue clothes and girls in pink, and also behaviours observed in the way parents soothe their babies may be in respect of their gender, for example, fathers being gentler when playing with their daughters (Schoppe-Sullivan *et al.* 2006). However, Schoppe-Sullivan *et al.* (2006) concede that when mother–male bonding is deficient, fathering takes on a sensitive and nurturing role.

This societal behaviour is supported by social learning theory; reasoning that girls and boys behave differently because they are treated differently from birth. Bandura (1977) brought attention to this model of human behaviour in the presence of continuous interactions and environmental influences. Bandura observed that the processes underlying learning through observation are described by four distinct features: attention, retention, motor reproduction and motivation.

Putting this into a framework for the purpose of parenthood and gender, a female child that behaves as its mother will receive praise and reinforcement of her behaviour; she identifies that this is good and that her continued role-play will be enhanced for future approval. This theory has some criticisms, for example, small boys who enjoy female pursuits cannot be disputed; however, parents and significant carers have a critical role to play in how their offspring behave. There is no doubt that the gender of the child influences parenting.

Fathering – new man or rightful role?

The role of the father is less than fairly represented in literature, particularly in the early work of Bowlby who based much of his primary observations on maternal relationships with their infants (Bowlby 1969). However, he was to clarify this later; 'almost from the first, many children have more than one attachment figure towards whom they direct attachment behaviour; these figures are not treated alike; the role of the child's principal attachment figure can be filled by others than the natural mother … It is evident that whom a child selects as his principal attachment figure and to how many other figures he becomes attached, turn in large part on who cares for him and on the composition of the household in which he is living.'

Explaining the role of the father has gained force over the last few decades; initially, most social scientists doubted that fathers significantly shaped the experiences and development of their children, especially their daughters. Research in this area has mainly focused upon three regions, that fathers

- have a role to play in a child's development;
- are salient in their child's life;
- influence the course of their children's lives for both good and bad effect.

Lamb *et al.* (1985) identified that fathers have more commonly been associated with play rather than in the caretaking role more often fulfilled by mothers. In fact research has identified that those men who believe they should be involved in the day-to-day caregiving of children, are more likely to be considered non-traditional in their principles. Allen and Hawkins (1999) describe the role of involved fathers sabotaged by 'maternal gate keeping'; the mother who tends to all of her child's needs and allows the father to contribute in a very specific or minor way.

Over the last three decades, fathers have been encouraged to access their pregnancies in more substantial ways. Maternity services have opened their doors to receive men into their once female-only environment; parent education programmes have more or less insisted that fathers attend and perhaps made to feel guilty if they are not in the birthing room (Buist *et al.* 2003). Midwifery practices have even changed to engage fathers, with offers of cutting the cord and actively participating in labour support.

Enkin *et al.* (2000) acknowledge that fathers today have an important and dynamic role in the birth process: they are encouraged to reinforce childbirth education principles, act as advocates for the mother, and support the woman in her labour and postnatal recovery. The interdependent behaviour of both mother and father is complex; this dynamic will influence outcomes on the following:

- Breastfeeding
- Maternal mental well-being
- Resuming sexual relationships
- Smoking
- Confidence and skills in parenting (Fischer 2007).

The Department of Health and other professional bodies have acknowledged the part that fathers play in pregnancy and parenthood, real engagement of fathers is critical not only to the outcome of the birth experience but also in the way a new family is established. The Fatherhood Institute working with Fathers Direct identifies the changing role of fatherhood; 'fifty years ago few fathers in Britain attended the birth of their baby. Now 86% of all fathers attend the birth – 95% of parents who live together are together for the birth and the same is true of 45% of parents who live apart. No health or family service other than maternity achieves remotely this level of connection in their role as carers of children' (Fischer 2007).

The benefit of working more closely with fathers has been identified with positive outcomes for both mother and child. 'Involvement of prospective and new fathers in a child's life is extremely important for maximising the life-long well-being and outcomes of the child (regardless of whether the father is resident or not). Pregnancy and birth are the first major opportunities to engage fathers in appropriate care and upbringing of children' (Department of Health 2004).

Fathers who are less likely to be involved in maternity services in a meaningful way and experience prejudice are young fathers. Fischer (2007) states that too often young fathers are described as 'hard to reach' but this is often because services are not creative when trying to reach them. The implications of excluding young fathers is significant, young men who become fathers are more likely to be living in disadvantaged social circumstances and may have to deal with stigma such as being disinterested in fathering.

There is no doubt that a child needs both parents, empirical evidence supports this. Both mother and a father bring their own unique characteristics to the family relationship; and ultimately influence the future well-being and potential of their child. Maternity services have a mandate to care for both mother and father, ensuring that neither is mutually exclusive. While this might be a challenge for maternity, the future of the couple as parents will no doubt be enhanced by good quality care that is respectful of the importance of the family as a unit.

The final transition to parenthood

The confirmation of pregnancy, morning sickness, anxiety about screening tests and final hurdle of labour to bring the infant to meet its parents is a lengthy journey that midwives share with families.

Women are the focus, they are making the physical, emotional and psychological leaps 'From Me to Mother' (Gutteridge 2002) some manage with ease, others struggle and take a long period of adjustment. The stories and truths women describe after their childbearing experiences are a rich fount of information; we need these narratives to both understand the quality of care and also build pathways that are respectful and responsive.

Understanding how women think and reach a level of achievement as mothers is complex and unique; it will even change from child to child. Her experiences as a daughter will be the template of her future parenting; she will accept and reject practices from her own parents. The influence of society has the potential to mould and lead trends in childbearing and motherhood, it is vital to understand these sociological nuances.

Midwives are part of the journey that women make into their unknown, they can support, educate, advocate and influence the outcomes, and their position is powerful and undisputed. The way midwives and maternity services engage with fathers and other family members are critical, women generally need to feel their families are welcomed and inclusive.

The relationships women have with their developing fetuses starts very early in the pregnancy and cements throughout with factors such as screening and fetal movements influencing this unique union. Her dreams are more vivid, her fantasies extreme reinforcing her fears and aspirations of both her baby and also her own potential as a mother. The closeness she experiences in the first few minutes after birth affirms her bonding with her baby and her dreams finally becoming reality.

To be part of this journey is a privilege, it should not be undertaken lightly and treated with the respect and nurturance it deserves, for the future of the child with its parents is part of our service.

Key implications for midwifery practice

- The experience of pregnancy is unique for each woman. Consider how women you care for are adjusting to the physical, psychological and emotional changes of pregnancy. Ask them how they are feeling and how they are coping with being pregnant.
- Physical contact with a newborn baby is important for all mothers. Consider how you support this practice for all women in different circumstances. You might want to explore new ways of working to ensure that mothers have the opportunity to see and be with their baby at all times.
- Fathers are an important part of a baby's life, providing support and care to both the new baby and its mother. Consider how you support the needs of the father throughout pregnancy, the birth and beyond. You might want to look at how your maternity service meets the needs of fathers and families.

References

Affleck G, Tennen H (1991) The effect of newborn intensive care on parents' psychological well-being. *Child Health Care* 20: 6–14.

Ainsworth MDS, Blehar MC, Waters E, Wall S (1978) *Patterns of Attachment: A Psychological Study of the Strange Situation*. Hillsdale, NJ: Erlbaum.

Allen SM, Hawkins AJ (1999) Maternal gatekeeping: Mothers' beliefs and behaviors that inhibit greater father involvement in family work. *Journal of Marriage and Family* 61: 199–212.

Baillie C, Hewison J, Mason G (1996) The Psychological potential of routine ultrasound scanning: a systematic review of the evidence. *Journal of Reproductive and Infant Psychology* 14: 324.

Bandura A (1977) *Social Learning Theory*. New York: General Learning Press.

Benassi L, Accorsi F, Marconi L, Benassi G (2004) Psychobiology of the amniotic environment. *Acta Bio Medica Ateneo Parmense* 75 (Suppl. 1): 18–22.

Bornstein MH (1989) Sensitive periods in development: structural characteristic and causal interpretations. *Psychological Bulletin* 105: 179–197.

Bowlby J (1951) *Maternal Care and Mental Health, Monograph Serial No. 2*. London: World Health Organization.

Bowlby J (1969) *Attachment and Loss, Attachment*, Vol. 1. London: Pelican.

Buist A, Morse CA, Durkin S (2003) Men's adjustment to fatherhood: implications for obstetric health care. *Journal of Obstetric, Gynecologic, and Neonatal Nursing* 32 (2): 172–180, ISSN: 0884-2175.

Chodorow N (1978) *The Reproduction of Mothering*. Berkeley and Los Angeles: University of California Press.

Clement S, Wilson J, Sikorski J (1998) Women's experiences of antenatal ultrasound scans. In: Clement S (ed). *Psychological Perspectives on Pregnancy and Childbirth*. London: Churchill Livingstone.

De Casper AJ, Fifer WP (1980) Of human bonding: newborns prefer their mothers' voices. *Science* 208: 1174–1176.

Department of Health (2004) *National Service Framework for Children, Young People and Maternity Services Standard 11*. London.

Enkin MW, Kierse MJNC, Neilson J, *et al.* (2000) *A Guide to Effective Care In Pregnancy and Childbirth*, 3rd Edition. Oxford: Oxford University Press.

Field T, Diego M, Hernandez-Reif M (2006) Prenatal depression effects on the fetus and newborn: a review. *Infant Behavior and Development* 29 (3): 445–455.

Fischer D (2007) *Information Leaflet–Including New Fathers, A Guide for Maternity Professionals*, available at www.fathersdirect.com (accessed 18/03/2008).

Forna A (1998) *Mother of all Myths–How Society Moulds and Constrains Mothers*. London: Harper Collins.

Freud S (1926) Inhibitions, symptoms and anxiety. *Standard Edition of the Complete Psychological Works of Sigmund Freud*, Vol. 20. London: Hogarth Press.

Freud S (1940a) *An Outline of Psycho-Analysis*, Vol. 23: 141–207. London: Hogarth Press.

Freud S (1940b) *Splitting of the Ego in the Process of Defence*, Vol. 23: 273–278. London: Hogarth Press.

Gerhardt S (2004) *Why Love Matters*. London: Routledge.

Gutteridge KEA (2002) *From Me To Mother–A Descriptive Phenomenological Exploration of Women's' Journey into Motherhood Informed by Feminist Theory*. Unpublished thesis for MSc Counselling and Psychotherapy University of Central England.

Kagan J (1978) *The Growth of the Child*. New York: Norton.

Kitzinger S (2005) *The Politics of Birth*. London: Elsevier.

Klaus MH, Kennell JH (1976) Parent to infant attachment. In: Hull A (eds). *Recent Advances in Paediatrics*, Vol. 5. New York: Churchill Livingstone.

Klein M (1998) *Love, Guilt and Reparation: and Other Works*. London: Vintage.

Lamb ME (1978) Qualitative aspects of mother-infant and father-infant attachments in the second year of life. *Infant Behavior and Development* 1: 265–275.

Lamb ME, Pleck JH, Levine JA (1985) The role of the father in child development: the effects of increased paternal involvement. In: Lahey BB, Kazdin AE (eds). *Advances in Clinical Child Psychology*, Vol. 8. New York: Plenum, 229–266.

Lieberman E, Torday J, Barbieri R, Cohen A, Van Vunakin H, Weiss ST (1992) Association of intrauterine cigarette smoke exposure with indices of fetal lung maturation. *Obstetrics and Gynecology* 79: 564–570.

Lorenz KZ (1935) Der Kumpan in der Vmwalt des Vogels. *Journal of Ornithology*. Reprinted in Schiffer CH (1957) (ed.). *Instinctive Behaviour*. Methuen.

Maslow AW (1943) A theory of human motivation. *Psychological Review* 50: 370–396.

Niven CA (1992) *Psychological Care for Families: Before, During and After Birth*. Oxford: Butterworth Heinemann.

Odent M (1978) The fetus ejection reflex. *Birth* 14: 104–105.

Odent M (1991) Fear of death during labour. *Journal of Reproductive and Infant Psychology* 9: 43–47.

Raphael-Leff J (2001) *Psychological Processes of Childbearing*, revised edition. London: Chapman & Hall.

Rose A (1992) Effects of childhood sexual abuse on childbirth: one woman's story. *Birth* 19 (44): 214–218.

Rutter M (1981) *Maternal Deprivation Reassessed*, 2nd Edition. Harmondsworth: Penguin.

Schaffer HR, Emerson PK (1964) The development of social attachments in infancy. *Monographs of the Society for Research in Child Development* 29 (serial 94).

Schoppe-Sullivan SJ, Diener ML, Mangelsdorf SC, Brown GL, McHale JL, Frosch CA (2006) Attachment and sensitivity in family context: the roles of parent and infant gender. *Infant and Child Development* 15 (4): 367–385.

Sered S, Abramovitch H (1992) Pregnant dreaming: searching for a typology of a proposed dream genre. *Social Science and Medicine* 34 (12): 1405–1411.

Simkin P (1991) Just another day in a woman's life? Women's long-term perceptions of their first birth experience. *Birth* 18 (4): 203–210.

Winnicott DW (1957) *Mother and Child. A Primer of First Relationships*. New York: Basic Books, Inc.

Wolf N (2001) *Misconceptions; Truth, Lies and Unexpected on the Journey to Motherhood*. London: Chatto & Windus Publishers.

Chapter 5
Empowering Mothers: Strengthening the Future

Sheena Byrom and Anna Gaudion

Involving women and families

The National Health Service (NHS) in the United Kingdom is pursuing every possible opportunity to fully engage with communities and individuals in the design and delivery of its services. Efforts are being made to ask people for their views about their experience of services; to contribute to staff training, to national policy and to be members of NHS foundation trusts. NICE (2008) has developed guidance on community engagement, and the document highlights the fact that using approaches to help communities to work as equal partners, and delegate power to them, may lead to positive health outcomes. Providing opportunities for the views and opinions of local people to be heard is encouraged so that decisions and developments will potentially be better informed. There is also a commitment for the engagement and empowerment of communities to be a mainstream activity in the commissioning of services. This agenda provides some opportunity for midwives and mothers (and fathers) to work together to improve maternity services in general, but also, and significantly more importantly, to influence health and social gain within families, and populations.

There has been much debate about the power relationships between midwives and obstetricians (Donnison 1998; Mander 2004), midwives and midwives (Curtis *et al.* 2006; Bird 2007) and midwife and mother (Pairman 2000). Within each discussion, empowerment of the woman during the childbirth process has been the focus. The fundamental, optimal partnership between mother and midwife is profound and the consequences of the liaison between the two have been described as triumphant or tragic (Kitzinger 2006; Thomson 2007). This chapter will explore how simple positive connections between mother and midwife can build trust and confidence that results in women feeling able to positively engage with their child, family and community. This chapter will explore the fact that the impact of empowerment is far reaching; a model of midwifery care that facilitates and encourages knowledge sharing as opposed to one that fosters dependence and reliance, maximises potential for mothers and fathers to feel confident and positive, and enhances the potential for life-changing activities.

The midwife–mother relationship and the postnatal period

Chapter 1 of this book eloquently highlights the history and important significance of the education and professionalisation of midwifery within the United Kingdom, in relation to improving health outcomes for mothers and babies in the postnatal period. The chapter cites specific textbooks that promoted activities that reduced risk of morbidity and mortality following childbirth, rather than focusing on recovery and return to normal health. Today, some of the practices outlined in these books continue to exist, and current surveillance and monitoring of both mother and infant from the moment of birth necessitates activities from many healthcare workers, including midwives, heathcare assistants, obstetricians, paediatricians, anaesthetists, health visitors, hearing screening coordinators and GPs. When this 'support' or 'treatment' ceases, the woman is potentially at risk of feeling isolated, especially when family and friends are absent (Leap 2000). Leap (2000) warns midwives not to foster mutually dependant relationships, but to encourage women to tap into social support; to guide them into building a network around them to counteract seclusion following birth.

For many women, childbirth is a pivotal event in their lives. In 1997, Belenky *et al.* reported on an in-depth qualitative study of 'women's ways of knowing'. When women were asked what the most important learning experience they had had in their lives, many selected childbirth. Ann said:

> My life was really, really dull. The only thing that really stands out is the birth of my children. That's the only thing that has happened to me ever. So that's about it.
>
> (Belenky *et al.* 1997, p. 35)

This mother [Ann], being vulnerable, needed support in parenting and accessed 'the experts' to help her. Ann describes how they succeeded by emphasising *her* competence, not theirs, which in turn gave her confidence and courage to 'tame the world'. In this instance, the health worker held the ingredient for change, and gave the 'power' away to Ann thus influencing her behaviour and confidence, which resonated throughout her family. But then the process of empowerment went one step further. Ann described how not only did she receive knowledge from her supporters, but was able to share it, and she became the expert amongst her friends (Belenky *et al.* 1997). In her chapter, 'The less we do the more we give', Leap (2000) prompts midwives to promote women's awareness and sense of independence and responsibility. Leap describes this as a process of inspiring confidence in women and encourages midwives to positively affirm the woman's courage and abilities following the birth, which may increase her ability to engage in the empowering process of reflection in the early postnatal period.

Leap (2000) also suggests that in the postnatal period it is far more beneficial clinically, and for the women's esteem, to ask a woman how her baby is rather than 'strip searching' him to check, thus undermining the mothers ability to know. The author also debates the negative process of 'top to toe' checking of the mother, with the undignified 'checking the pad', and encourages listening to women and only performing such checks if the mother raises concerns. These proposals are affirmed in recommendations made by NICE in their guidelines for postnatal care (NCCPC 2006), which place emphasis on self-care and knowledge, in contrast to routine checking:

> Women should be offered relevant and timely information to enable them to promote their own and their babies' health and well-being and to recognise and respond to problems.
>
> (NCCPC 2006)

Promoting and supporting women to take responsibility for their own or their baby's health will positively encourage women to make choices. Through sourcing the information to assist them, sometimes women will potentially make choices that don't 'fit' with a professional view point and are deemed as a 'risk'.

Choice and risk: who knows best?

In the United Kingdom, healthcare workers are encouraged to achieve Lord Darzi's vision (Department of Health 2007a) for an NHS that is:

> personalised – tailored to the needs and wants of each individual, especially the most vulnerable and those in greatest need.

The direction is backed up by medical and midwifery professional legislation (General Medical Council 2006; Nursing and Midwifery Council (NMC) 2008), and several NICE clinical guidelines related to maternity care[1]. Increasing availability of information technology systems provides an enhanced opportunity for women to access knowledge in relation to childbirth. The NHS is driving the choice agenda[2] in all areas of health care, including maternity (Department of Health 2007b, 2008), and yet for this service, the rhetoric is that 'choice' is frequently dependant on the provider of services, both at an individual and organisational level. The subject of informed choice has been debated by experts and researchers over many years (Kirkham 2004; Symon 2006; Jomeen 2007; Homeyard & Gaudion 2008), and in reality, it could be suggested that the hierarchical culture of NHS maternity care in general frequently hinders the process, especially when a woman's choice does not resonate with the beliefs or knowledge of her caregiver. If midwives strive to remember that woman-centred care and 'choice' is when all parties acknowledge the facts, and the women then lead the decision, they are maximising potential for positive health outcomes. But frequently the mother's inherent knowledge of her own body is often diminished, and seen as less important than that of the healthcare worker/professional. When health professionals believe they know best, even when the mother thinks differently, the consequences are quite different and substantially damaging. Sue had been diagnosed as being Group B Strep positive in her first pregnancy, although her baby was not affected. And then:

> When I fell pregnant with my second daughter I became very interested in natural childbirth, more so than with my previous pregnancy, and decided that a home birth would give me the best chance of achieving a natural, drug free, birth. Because of my history of GBS I did a lot of research and decided not to be tested (as the test has a 50% false negative rate) and to go ahead with the homebirth I wanted, without antibiotics. Mainly this was because the transmission rate of GBS from mother to newborn seemed, in my opinion, to be low enough for the risk to be negligible (the highest I could find was 0.33%) I was worried that I would come up with opposition but my midwifery team were on the whole very supportive, once that had established that my decision was an informed one. We decided to swab the baby after delivery and I would observe the baby at home for signs of infection. I also declined a membrane sweep at 40 weeks and kept internal examination to a minimum as I had read of a theoretical risk to the fetus if the mother carried GBS.

Sue's home birth was straightforward, but shortly afterwards the baby developed rapid respirations and was transferred to the hospital. Medical staff wanted to perform a series of invasive procedures and blood tests were taken, in addition to the commencement of intravenous antibiotics.

I was 41 weeks pregnant, I didn't have a temperature during labour, and the duration of ROM was only 28 minutes. This, coupled with the fact that I hadn't actually tested positive for GBS this pregnancy and I haven't had a previous baby with a GBS infection reassured me, as I had no addition risk factors. However, my daughter's respiration rate was increased, and when the midwife called the paediatrician at the hospital for advice, we were transferred to the postnatal ward for (I thought) observation. I was upset to be separated from my partner and our other daughter but I didn't want to take any unnecessary risk with our new child. I arrived at the hospital at midnight; two doctors came to see us and examined my baby. Her respiration rate was now down to 66 (it was 80 at home) but there was a slight dipping below her ribs. I was not worried about her as she was pink, alert, active and feeding well (although I understand that GBS infection can begin later).

The doctors wanted to take her to NICU for a lumbar puncture, blood test and antibiotics. I was devastated at the thought of my 4 hour old daughter being separated from me and having such invasive procedures performed on her. I asked lots of questions from the doctors and called my partner for his opinion. We wanted to wait until the morning before deciding whether to allow the test. However, the doctors were not happy with this and after a lot of persuasion on the part of the doctors I agreed, at 4.30 am, that if my baby could stay on the ward with me she could have the blood cultures and antibiotics. The doctor seemed to accept that it was my decision but she got me to agree to the antibiotics by using 'scare tactics' I'm not uninformed and I am fully aware that babies die from GBS infection, I don't think it is necessary for the doctor to tell a vulnerable woman about the babies that she has seen die etc. from GBS. The doctor said that if it was her child she would defiantly give her the antibiotics – I suggested that as she was a doctor she was probably biased, as she always got to see the worse case scenario to which she replied, 'I am not biased, I am educated'.

This mother found these comments harrowing and totally disempowering. After 48 hours of antibiotics the baby's blood cultures showed no abnormal growth and Sue wanted to take her baby home. The baby had no symptoms and her respiration rate had been normal since that first night. The doctor came to see Sue and her partner and told them they needed to stay in overnight for observation as her CRPs were raised.

> My partner was not happy with this but we agreed. However, during the discussion with the doctor he said to my partner 'if she was my child I would stay in … I'm not saying you're bad parents but … ' We both found this really unprofessional and were offended by his judgement on our parenting.

The following day the doctor from the previous night came to see Sue and informed her that as the CRP levels were still elevated she needed to restart the antibiotics and the baby needed to remain in hospital for another 72 hours. Sue did not feel this was necessary as her baby was symptom-free, and was feeding well. She was very upset and called her partner to come, and whilst waiting for him to arrive agreed to another blood culture.

> I cried while my baby screamed as he [doctor] replaced her drip and took a blood sample. I was so upset as I felt the treatment she was receiving was unnecessary and I felt like a bad mother for not protecting her from the doctors when I knew that she didn't need to have this painful procedure done.

Sue and her partner decided eventually to decline further antibiotics and to go home. There was further negative communication with medical staff, although the midwife discussed our plan to go home and to return if the blood tests showed any deterioration. The doctor was not happy.

> After a while the doctor came to speak to us and outlined why he felt we should stay in. While I completely understood his position I felt he was very disrespectful to my partner and I. He wouldn't let my partner speak – he keep saying 'can you please let me finish' whenever my partner tried to raise an objection to what he was saying. We are intelligent people and we understood what the doctor was explaining to us – however, as we didn't agree that the treatment was necessary he assumed that we were missing something. He repeatedly said 'I don't feel like you've got all the information' – I genuinely think he couldn't see our point of view and assumed as we didn't agree with mustn't have all the information.
>
> When it became clear to him were weren't going to agree with him he started using 'scare tactics' he said to us 'I've seen babies who look fine one minute and they are dead within 6 hours.' He also said 'How would you feel if you take you baby home and she dies'?

I was already sobbing before he said this and I feel this was an awful thing to say to us and completely unprofessional – neither of these comments help us make an informed choice about treatment. He said to my partner 'I care about the baby – I don't care what you have to say all I care about is the baby' When he saw that we were not backing down he said that we had to wait to see the registrar and he would have to inform social services! The registrar did not come to see us as he/she said that as long as our decision was informed then we could go home. No one mentioned social services again.

The impact that this experience had on Sue is far reaching; and negatively affected her time as a new mother. She felt that she had let her baby down, a feeling other mothers frequently articulate when their newborn baby needs invasive treatment 'as a precaution'.

And from the minute we entered the hospital until the day we left I felt fully confident that she (baby) was fine and we didn't need to be there – I feel as though I have failed her because I wasn't strong enough to stand up for what I thought was best for her. If the doctors had listened to my opinion and respected my decision as her mother things would have been very different and I could have enjoyed the first two weeks of my daughters life.

It is clear from Sue's story that the doctors assumed 'expert' knowledge, and had 'power over' the mother and baby. They saw lack of compliance as lack of understanding and then used 'bullying' and scare tactics to try to change the decision, as described by Kirkham (2004). It appears the midwife played a somewhat background role in the story, albeit a more positive one, although it could be argued that there was no advocate for the parents. This is frequently the situation when 'risk' is deemed to be critical, and the medical team is articulating the 'certainty' of the consequences.

Sue's account is very different from one told by Worth (2008), in her memoirs of working as a midwife in the West End of London in the 1950s. Worth describes sensitively the details of the birth of Conchita and Len's twenty-fifth child, born early at around 28 weeks' gestation, at home. Labour had been 'induced' by a fall, and following the birth Conchita had a severe post-partum haemorrhage. The baby was thought to be dead at birth, but on realising the opposite, a call was made for assistance from Great Ormond St. The allocated team consisted of two doctors and a nurse, and added to the doctors and midwife already present in the bedroom, they proceeded to focus their attention on the baby. Conchita, who only spoke Spanish and was semi-conscious, had her hand on the baby and wouldn't let the paediatrician take him. More persuasion ensued from Conchita and Len's eldest child

Liz (who spoke Spanish) and the dramatic reaction from Conchita was startling:

> She [Conchita] opened her eyes wide, desperately trying to focus on the people around her. She saw the equipment and the white coats. I think her clouded brain took it all in, and she struggled to sit up. Liz and Len helped her. She looked wildly round at everyone, thrust the baby down between her breasts, and folded her arms over him. (p. 298)

There was then a debate from all parties as to the importance of taking the baby to the hospital. Liz softly told her mother in Spanish that the baby may die. But Conchita remained sure that the baby would die if he went, so refused to release him. Eventually Len stepped in, and told the medical team:

> This is all my fault and I must apologise. I said the baby could go, without consultin' my wife. I shouldn't 'ave done that. When it comes to the kiddies she must always have the last word, she must. An' she don't agree with it. You can see she don't, an' so the baby's not goin' nowhere. He'll stop 'ere with us, an he'll be christened, an' if he dies, he'll have a Christian burial. But he's not goin' nowhere without 'is mother's consent.

The story goes on, the baby survived, and Len had complete faith in Conchita, who told him the baby would not die. But the dialogue above demonstrates clearly where the power base lay; it was certainly with the mother. No threats of social services, no continued persuasion from the medical team. Len was an advocate for Conchita, and that was that.

The two scenarios have similar themes, and yet contrasting conclusions; we are sure from the story that Conchita did not feel she had allowed harm to come to her baby. The book is not explicit in whether or not Conchita was proud of her decision, but the reader can make a strong assumption that she probably was very proud indeed.

And what about women who are doubly vulnerable; through poverty or social circumstance? They too need and require respect and recognition that they are experts in their own social and lifestyle experiences. Women are aware if they are treated differently, be it because they are poor, are new migrants to the county, have particular problems such as mental health or addiction problems, or have previous children in care. A woman with a problematic addiction shared her perspective:

> I put it off, going I mean, till I was eight months gone. It was their attitude; therefore I put it off . . . it makes you afraid . . . they did not

want to know ... I mean the organic women, you know those ladies with partners and a bag packed, they get treated differently, they get asked not told.

(Homeyard & Gaudion 2008, p. 22)

A woman from Morocco described how the partnership model advocated in the National Service Framework and Maternity Matters (Department of Health 2004, 2007a) was not her experience:

A Ford factory mechanism, no informed consent ... no means of stopping the conveyor-belt ... not really worth me going, I got nothing out of it.

(Homeyard & Gaudion 2008, p. 22)

Midwives–mother relationship, community development and social capital

Pairman (2000) in her exploratory study of the relationship of mother and midwife describes how women bring to the partnership knowledge of their self and family and an expectation of trust and respect. With a background of professional and ethical standards, the midwife brings her ability to 'be with' women. From the study, Pairman (2000) suggests that women and midwives work together and uses words such as 'reciprocity', 'sharing power and control', 'building trust', 'being equal' to describe the process. Research conducted by the Polyanna Project (Gaudion *et al.* 2007b) highlighted the importance of kinship, friendships and trusted relationships in enabling women to access and use services effectively. Women do not rationalise becoming a parent as isolated events neatly partitioned by professional structures into antenatal, intrapartum and postnatal categories, but being a part of life (Gaudion 2007).

Community development is a concept that is more frequently utilised by health visitors than midwives. Health visitor education programmes encourage this model of care, to assist in the mobilisation of latent or undeveloped skills within a community and therefore enhancing potential for sustained change. However, midwives who work to deliver true woman-centred philosophies of care, will recognise that they are utilising the same underlying principles of community development philosophy, when they work in partnership, empowering and enabling the woman, and facilitating the childbirth process by engaging in a trusting relationship. Similarly, community development 'focuses on bringing people together, whilst empowering individuals. It is associated with the words "encourage" "facilitate" and "enable" "trust". Community development projects dependence back to individuals who may become community leaders themselves' (Health Development Agency 2004).

> Communities are wise, if you give us a choice and include and embrace our voices, allow us to bring forward our experiences and visions we can become doorways rather than divisions.
>
> (Gaudion *et al*. 2007a, p. 39)

Peer support could be identified as an example of community development, where individuals develop skills and knowledge, and then help others in a variety of ways. Midwives and mothers co-wrote a book chapter (Henry *et al*. 2007) on a peer support project relevant to maternity services, describing a group of local mothers who developed an idea for mother-to-mother support for breastfeeding, known as 'Little Angels'[3]. 'Little Angels' is a living example of community development – local mothers wanted to help other mothers, so learned new skills alongside and from health professionals, and continually share their knowledge within the communities they serve through support for breastfeeding. Midwives work in partnership with the peer supporters to develop and run the service, and together they have increased the knowledge base and capacity within an increasingly expanding community.

The success of this development is demonstrated in increased breastfeeding initiation and duration rates, but equally, with the positive impact on the peer supporter's lives:

> Kauser informed us that this was her first job. Her mother had a stroke and her husband had a heart attack. She was feeling depressed, then Little Angels offered her a job. Now she feels every day she is reborn.
>
> (Henry *et al*. 2007, p. 202)

See 5.1 for another practice example of community development.

Box 5.1 Example of community development

'Parents 1st' is a social enterprise that supports organisations to develop local and autonomous community-owned programmes focusing on early prevention. Community mothers, fathers or carers are advocates and intermediaries who complement and work alongside local professionals. The aim is to transfer skills to local communities enabling carefully recruited experienced parents to promote maternal and postnatal health, family well-being and early parenting skills within their own communities. A volunteer to employment training and progression pathway builds the capacity to self-deliver. Some experienced volunteers move into employment as support workers, health trainers or assistant coordinators.

The programmes include evidence-based, semi-structured home visiting, breastfeeding peer support and health literacy tuition. The empowerment model used is based on principles of mutual respect, self-help, avoiding dependency and focusing on solutions. Antenatal health needs assessments carried out by midwives and public health nurses provide important gateways for disadvantaged parents. Each peer outreach visit builds on the previous one, using listening and confidence-building skills to enable the gradual development of early coping skills. Parents self-select and achieve ongoing goals relevant to the context of their own daily lives. A wide range of health and early parenting outcomes have been demonstrated that span across the 'Every Child Matters' outcomes framework.

A research study (Suppiah 2008) of 10 programmes operating across the United Kingdom identified two critical ingredients for successful programmes. It is vital to select volunteers who have particular strengths, personal qualities and interpersonal skills. This ensures that trusting peer relationships are developed with marginalised parents, providing emotional support and enabling parents to access services. The other crucial ingredient is investing in skilled community development practitioners (level 6/7) with dedicated time to coordinate and develop local programmes. Their responsibilities are multifaceted such as ongoing supervision and personal development support for volunteers; ensuring safe operational boundaries are adhered to; providing ongoing high-quality accredited training; and embedding participatory evaluation. Effective delivery of these community development skills provides the foundations for successful programmes.

Empowering communities and increasing social capital

When considering the potential for increasing self-esteem of women during the childbirth continuum, midwives will become aware of the potential they hold for enhancing community confidence and knowledge. As described briefly earlier in this chapter, Ann (Belenky *et al.* 1997) increased her knowledge in relation to childcare and parenting, and then felt able to be the advisor and share conformance with her family and friends:

I now feel very knowledgeable as far as kids go. I advise all my friends with kids, you know. I say "this is what I've learned at the centre". I've learned a lot. I feel like I could go in there, and they could hire me, you know, that's how much knowledge they have given me.

Ann describes in real terms the process of increasing social capital. Social capital refers to 'the network and trust between people, which can be highly significant in building strong communities, combating social exclusion and providing a basis for long term economic development' (Health Development Agency 2004). When midwives work closely with women, sharing information and facilitating the liberation of internal assets, they are contributing to the growth of social capital.

An example of utilising community development approaches through positive connection can be demonstrated through Jane (mother) and Brenda's (midwife) story.

Brenda:

When I first met Jane [mother] she came to see me at a local community house, that was being used until the Children's Centre was built. Jane had complex family issues that contributed to her suffering from anxiety and stress. I remember she was very tearful and obviously distressed, I was concerned if I had the necessary skills to help her.

I felt that I needed to support Jane because she was vulnerable due to the fact that she thought she was in an inescapable circle of motherhood, depression and being unable to cope. The support I gave was listening visits but sometimes they would change to talking visits and part of caring is sharing a little of yourself so people you care for know you are human too.

It seemed to me that in no time at all L (baby) was born and Jane had to cope with hormonal changes and a new baby and breastfeeding. Jane had breastfed both of her older children, but felt she needed support so she came to the local group where she met lots of other local mums. Jane was so enthusiastic about breastfeeding and its benefits to both mum and baby that I just knew I had to have her on 'my team'. I was facilitating local breastfeeding mums to do a twelve week peer support course and Jane was in the first group to graduate. I constantly asked Jane for support and help as this seemed to light a spark in her somewhere. I was aware she still had issues with family but I hope I was always supportive and understanding when the going got tough.

Jane:

It's quite difficult for me to cast myself back to when things were so much different for me then. I was pregnant with my third child, and having previously suffered from depression, I was really scared of it returning. I had a lot of social problems and low self esteem, I felt I had failed as a parent before and didn't have much confidence in my abilities this time around.

I was put in touch with Brenda through Sure Start, and the first time I met her I think I cried for over an hour. I was a wreck emotionally and didn't see much of a future for myself. Brenda was so supportive and helpful; nothing was too much for her, she truly supported me in what is really my recovery, she made me feel important and always made herself available to me, especially after the birth of my daughter. She always had a smile and good advice. I had breastfed before but still needed my confidence building up. Brenda invited me to her baby massage group and breastfeeding group, and would even come and walk me down as I wasn't confident walking into a room alone. I slowly found myself able to get involved and chat to people, something I had found difficult before.

Brenda was facilitating the La Leche League Peer Support Counsellor training locally and asked if I would like to be involved. I agreed to be on the first group of mums to do the training and really enjoyed it. I was thrilled to be in a position to help other local mums and I knew I wanted to go up onto the postnatal wards at although there were some hurdles, we overcame them. I worked as a breastfeeding support volunteer for almost two years and am now employed by Little Angels, a Social Enterprise breastfeeding peer support company, as a breastfeeding supporter, doing a job that I truly love, supporting local mums to successfully breastfeed.

I have also trained and participated in research in partnership with midwives, health visitors and the local university, and have established a service user group for the development of birth centres.

I received funding to become a Doula, as I want to support women in pregnancy and labour, and to empower women. I know how much having a baby can really change you life and your outlook on life, and I want to share my enthusiasm and passion. I consider Brenda to be one of my closest friends; she is a very special person who made a huge difference in my life. She helped me to see a future and to believe in myself.

Jane now has confidence and skills to share with many others, which in turn has the potential to have a positive effect on her family, and the wider community, thereby increasing social capital.

See Box 5.2 for a practice example of improving social capital.

Box 5.2 Example of promoting social capital

In 2009, Kings College University Hospital will be piloting an innovative way of providing antenatal care which encourages and promotes social capital. The model of care is called 'Centering Pregnancy' and has been extensively rolled out in America. It involves women having their care in a group, rather than individually. Women are encouraged to be active participants in their care, The group sessions are semi-structured and facilitate discussions around a range of issues such as diet, expectations around birth, breastfeeding in accordance with the women's needs. Topics may also be sensitive such as domestic abuse, sexual health and depression (Schindler-Rising 1998). These topics are often more enabled in a group discussion which can be more general, and facilitate women to talk in the third person (Gaudion *et al.* 2008). One of the major advantages of this model of care is that women can learn from one another, it helps to build communities and enables support and problem-solving. Support develops naturally as the women develop friendships that continue long after the group has disbanded. In 'Centering Pregnancy' it is assumed that the woman is an expert about what she needs and knows, not the professional. The midwives have an important role to facilitate the flow of discussion, and by doing so, capitalise on the strengths and needs within the group (Schindler-Rising 1998).

'Centering Pregnancy', aims to tap into and encourage social capital and support with the hope that friendships made in the antenatal period will continue in the postnatal period. Social capital and health care are intertwined in this model of care with the women at the centre, which focuses on information sharing and engendering confidence in new mothers.

Revisions to the way that antenatal care is delivered, in groups rather than one-to-one, particularly to vulnerable groups has been shown to impact on postnatal outcomes. One randomised control study conducted in two US states recruited 1047 women and found that there was a significant reduction in the risk of prematurity by 33% (this risk reduction was greater for Afro-American women); increased breastfeeding initiation rates (Ickovics *et al.* 2007) and a significant increase in mean birth weight (Ickovics *et al.* 2003).

And for the future?

postnatal care is acknowledged as being under-resourced and fragmented. It could therefore seem an impossible task for midwives to spend extra time 'developing communities' or building social capital. However, these approaches to care mirror the philosophy of woman-centred care, which is a fundamental requirement within maternity services and should not be viewed as a desired option. Midwives have a 'magic moment' of opportunity that is relatively short but concentrated, where they can assist in building a woman's confidence through the words they use, and the position they set themselves. Working in the community, delivering care in Children Centres, community halls, churches and mosques, and being part of open days makes it easier for midwives to be visible and known. In addition, working with relevant voluntary and statutory agencies enhances the ability to provide consistent information and ensures that opportunities to engage and support women and families is facilitated.

For midwives and healthcare workers within maternity services, it is important to strive to promote an empowering facilitative model of care, wherever that care takes place, where the woman and her family is seen as true partners in ensuring their own health and future. If done well, the consequences have the potential to influence the mother's esteem, the mother–infant dyad, the mother–partner relationship and the baby's life, forever more.

Key implications for midwifery practice

- Has your maternity service implemented the recommendations from NICE postnatal Care guidelines, especially in relation to the promotion of self-care?
- If a woman 'declines' an intervention or treatment, is she supported or made to feel guilty?
- Do you really think about the words you use? Do you 'teach' mothers, or do you share your knowledge?
- If a woman or her family is unhappy with the care or complains, try to think about how they can help you to put things right. How can they get involved?
- Do you know how to signpost women for social support, and promote engagement with support networks?
- Do mothers have the opportunity to help other mothers in your unit? If not, how could you help to make it happen?
- Do local women in your area share their skills with others, such as breastfeeding?

Notes

1 http://www.nice.org.uk/
2 Web site dedicated to choice: www.nhs.uk/Pages/homepage.aspx
3 www.littleangels.org.uk/

References

Belenky MF, Clinchy BMc, Goldberger NR, Tarule JM (1997) *Women's Ways of Knowing: The Development of Self Voice and Mind*, 10th Anniversary Edition. New York: Basic Books.

Bird M (2007) Our own worst enemies. *Practising Midwife* 10 (5): 66.

Curtis P, Ball L, Kirkham M (2006) Bullying and horizontal violence: cultural or individual phenomena? *British Journal of Midwifery* 14 (4): 218–221.

Department of Health (2004) *The National Service Framework for Children, Young People and Maternity Services, Standard 11.* London: HMSO.

Department of Health (2007a) *Our NHS, Our Future,* October 2007.

Department of Health (2007b) *Maternity Matters: Choice, Access and Continuity of Care in a Safe Service.*

Department of Health (2008) *High Quality Care for All: NHS Next Stage Review Final Report,* Darzi.

Donnison J (1998) *Midwives and Medical Men: A History of the Struggle for the Control of Childbirth,* 2nd Edition. London: Historical Publications.

Gaudion A (2007) *The Development of the Maternity Access and Advocacy Pack,* available at: http://www.thepolyannaproject.org.uk/what-we-do.html.

Gaudion A, Godfrey C, Homeyard C, Cutts H (2007a) *The Hackney Women's Wheel Report,* available at: http://www.thepolyannaproject.org.uk/resources/wheel_report.pdf.

Gaudion A, Godfrey C, Homeyard C, Cutts H (2007b) *The Hackney Women's Wheel Visual Diary,* available at: http://www.thepolyannaproject.org.uk/resources/wheel_visual_diary.pdf.

Gaudion A, Godfrey C, Homeyard C, Cutts H (2008) *The Barking and Dagenham Women's Wheel Report,* available at: http://www.thepolyannaproject.org.uk/resources/barking_and_dagenham_report.pdf.

General Medical Council (2006) *Good Medical Practice.*

Health Development Agency (2004) *Developing Healthier Communities,* available at: www.nice.org.uk:80/aboutnice/whoweare/aboutthehda/hdapublications/hda_publications.jsp?o=538 (accessed 08/07/08).

Henry S, Dykes F, Byrom S, Atkin M, Jackson E (2007) Supporting breastfeeding: midwives facilitating a community model. In: Edwards G, Byrom S (eds). *Essential Midwifery Practice: Public Health.* Oxford: Blackwell Publishing.

Homeyard C, Gaudion A (2008) Safety in maternity services: women's perspectives. *The Practicing Midwife* 11 (7): 20–23.

Ickovics J, Kershaw T, Westdahl C, Magriples U, Schlinder-Rising S (2007) Group prenatal and perinatal outcomes. A randomised controlled trial. *Obstetrics and Gynaecology* 110: 330–339.

Ickovics J, Kershaw T, Westdahl C, Rising S, Klima C, Magriples U (2003) Group Prenatal care improves preterm birth weight: results from a matched cohort study at public clinics. *Obstetrics and Gynaecology* 102: 1051–1057.

Jomeen J (2007) Choice in childbirth: a realistic expectation? *British Journal of Midwifery* 15 (8): 485–490.

Kirkham M (2004) *Informed Choice in Maternity Care.* Basingstoke: Palgrave Macmillan.

Kitzinger S (2006) *Birth Crisis.* Oxon: Routledge Press.

Leap N (2000) The less we do, the more we give. In: Kirkham M (ed). *The Midwife–Mother Relationship.* London: Macmillan Press.

Mander R (2004) The midwife and medical men. In: Mander R (ed). *Men and Maternity.* London: Routledge.

National Institute of Clinical Excellence (2006) *Routine Postnatal Care of Women and their Babies*. National Collaborating Centre for Primary Care.

National Institute of Clinical Excellence (2008) *Community Engagement*, London.

Nursing and Midwifery Council (2008) *The Code-Standards of Conduct, Performance and Ethics for Nurses and Midwives*. London: NMC.

Pairman S (2000) Partnerships or professional friends? In: Kirkham M (ed). *The Midwife–Mother Relationship*. London: Macmillan Press.

Schindler-Rising S (1998) Centering pregnancy. An interdisciplinary model of empowerment. *Journal of Nurse-Midwife* 43 (1): 46–54.

Suppiah C (2008) *A Collective Evaluation of Community Mothers Programmes*. Research Report. South West Essex Primary Care Trust and The Health Foundation, available at: www.parents1st.org.uk.

Symon A (2006) *Risk and Choice in Maternity Care*. Edinburgh: Churchill Livingstone.

Thomson G (2007) *A Hero's Tale of Childbirth: An Interpretive Phenomenological Study of Traumatic and Positive Childbirth*. Unpublished thesis.

Worth J (2008) *Call the Midwife*. London: Orion Books.

Chapter 6
Morbidity during the Postnatal Period: Impact on Women and Society

Maria Helena Bastos and Christine McCourt

Introduction

Giving birth is usually a healthy process that is a part of women's normal lives, and is a major life event with biological, emotional and socio-cultural consequences. Childbirth should be understood as a bio-psychosocial process (Jordan 1993) which requires attention to all its complex effects on women's lives and well-being. While it is important to remember that the majority of women experience healthy pregnancies and with appropriate support will have straightforward births (MCWP 2008), childbirth is a challenging life event on many levels, and it is common for women to experience a range of problems post-natally. Commonly experienced problems range from fatigue and difficulty in adjusting to the demands of new motherhood to physical symptoms such as backache, pain from stitches and urinary incontinence.

In this chapter, we argue that it is very common for women to experience a number of postnatal health problems. Knowledge of this may reassure many women that their experiences are 'normal', but the impact on women's well-being also needs to be taken seriously by midwives and other healthcare professionals, with sufficient, appropriate support and information offered to women. postnatal morbidity, both physical and psychological, may have major long-term impacts on maternal and infant health. While this is challenging, particularly for hard-pressed staff in busy health services, it also forms an important opportunity for midwives and other healthcare providers to make a positive difference to public health at a key point of transition. Midwives may make a difference to health both by preventing morbidity and by responding effectively to the problems that women do experience.

Women's health and well-being are complex issues and different aspects are closely intertwined, but postnatal morbidity can be divided, analytically at least, into physical and psychosocial problems. When separating out such categories, however, we argue that it is important to remember how closely they are tied together in reality. Physical symptoms such as pain, for example, may impact on rest or fatigue and on psychological well-being; social factors such as level or type of support available may impact on the experience of pain and ability to recover from physical consequences of birth. This chapter outlines the different types of postnatal morbidity, and then focuses more closely on three key aspects of postnatal morbidity that are growing in significance in 'Western' countries: the consequences of Caesarean sections, the impact of perineal trauma and mental health problems following pregnancy and birth. Our focus on Caesarean sections is in response to the considerable rise in rates of operative birth in many countries in recent years. Despite Caesarean birth rates of over 30% in a number of countries, there has been very little emphasis in research or practice on the implications for postnatal health. Similarly, many practices relating to postnatal perineal care remain un-researched, and therefore, the impact on the woman's quality of life remains poorly understood. Our choice to focus on psychological health is based on two arguments; first, there is evidence that health care, post-natally, tends to focus on basic physical checks, paying limited attention to psychological well-being (WHO 1998; MacArthur *et al.* 2002, 2003); second, there is growing evidence that mental health problems can have a major impact on the long-term well-being of mothers and their families (Lewis 2004, 2007).

What is normal? The woman's perspective

With increasing social and geographical mobility, reduced family size and changing norms of work in modern and post-modern society, many women approach the birth of a first baby with relatively limited direct experience of pregnancy, birth, breastfeeding or childcare. The following quote, from a study of women's postnatal care experiences (Beake *et al.* 2005), illustrates the needs for basic support that may arise:

> I mean it's my first baby I didn't know anything you know, I mean they could have showed me how to change a nappy.

The average age of childbearing is higher, and the increasing proportion of women for whom pregnancy is planned may anticipate their baby's birth, with some trepidation, but also expectations of a healthy and fulfilling experience of new parenthood (McCourt & Beake 2001).

However, many women, when interviewed post-natally about their experiences, recount this as a difficult as well as joyful transition, and report many physical and psychological symptoms of ill-health rather than well-being (Bick & MacArthur 1995; Beck 2002; McCourt 2006). A number also lack practical knowledge and experience, increasing their needs for support (Beake *et al*. 2005). A number of commentators have also argued that pregnancy, birth and motherhood are becoming increasingly idealised in modern society, while at the same time more traditional sources of support are being eroded, so that women may feel stressed and disappointed by the realities of adjustment to parenthood (Barclay *et al*. 1997; Miller 2002; Abraham 2004; McCourt 2006). Additionally, a number of women experience pregnancy and birth in difficult social and economic circumstances, and there is clear evidence that they are particularly likely to suffer from health problems in pregnancy and after the birth (Hodnett & Fredericks 2007; Lewis 2007). Government enquiry reports on maternal and infant death in the United Kingdom have shown, for example, that in addition to difficult social circumstances, poor communication and liaison around care, problems of access to maternity services and problems in following through the healthcare system are all implicated in rates of death, as well as morbidity (Lewis 2004, 2007).

As childbirth itself has shifted from the largely domestic arena of birth at home to hospital birth in the late twentieth century in most resource-rich countries, social and family life has also undergone changes influencing the sources and kinds of support available to women following birth. Social networks and family ties are often highly geographically dispersed, and rates of mobility are high (McCourt 2009). A considerable proportion of women are in employment until late in pregnancy and sources of ordinary social support may be limited. The need for support from midwives has not diminished (Mander 2001).

Postnatal morbidity

Given the importance of postnatal health, surprisingly few studies have focused specifically on this aspect of women's experience. Additionally, few have attempted to assess general levels of morbidity, physically or psychologically, from women's perspectives. In the year following birth, 9 in 10 women will experience at least one major health problem. Most commonly reported physical morbidities are back pain, urinary or faecal incontinence, perineal pain, intercourse problems, breast problems, haemorrhoids, constipation and headaches (Bick & MacArthur 1995). Some health problems, such as perineal pain and incontinence, are more closely associated with the delivery itself, although others such as backache or headache are probably linked more to the increased demands of child care (MacArthur *et al.* 2003). The immediate concerns of postnatal care are with potentially life-threatening or serious morbidity, but many problems are long-term, and even when minor, they can have a significant impact on some aspects of the lives and well-being of women and their families (Bick & MacArthur 1995). A persistent finding of most studies in the United Kingdom is that many women do not report their postnatal problems to health professionals both in the earlier postnatal care period and later, despite the symptoms sometimes persisting for at least a year. Regardless of the availability of services, only half of the affected women sought treatment in the first year after birth, with even lower consultation rates for abnormal bleeding (44%), abdominal wound (19%), breastfeeding problems (41%), depression (59%), other psychological problems (46%), fatigue (21%), backache (30%), headache (17%), perineal pain/dyspareunia (39%), urinary symptoms (19%) or bowel symptoms (36%) (MacArthur *et al.* 2003). Reluctance to seek help was not because of limited contact with services, as availability and accessibility of home visits soon after hospital discharge by a health professional is universal in the United Kingdom.

In one of the few large-scale studies focused on women's postnatal morbidity in the United Kingdom, MacArthur *et al.* (2002) found that 47% of women reported health problems lasting more than 6 weeks and many lasted longer. Similarly, Glazener *et al.* (1995) found that 76% of women experienced at least one health problem between hospital discharge and the eighth postnatal week. Similarly, a large-scale survey in Australia (Brown & Lumley 1998, 2000) found that physical and emotional health problems are frequently not reported to health professionals despite the fact that many women would like more advice and assistance in dealing with them. In addition to physical symptoms, psychological problems such as depression have been found to be common post-natally (estimated by a wide range of studies to be present in at least 10–15% of women (Robertson *et al.* 2004; Leigh & Milgrom 2008)).

During the 1990s in the United Kingdom, a large study designed to evaluate a new model of midwifery care, following Changing Child-birth (Department of Health 1993), included a survey that asked women to report the type and levels of postnatal symptoms they were experiencing at 2 and 12 weeks following birth (McCourt & Page 1996). The study included women of all obstetric and social risk levels, who were receiving either caseload midwifery or the usual system of shared maternity care, depending on which part of a maternity service's local catchment area they lived in. The findings indicated that many women experienced a wide range of symptoms, and for some these were relatively severe and enduring. For example, over half of the women reported suffering backaches at 2 weeks post-natally, and at 12 weeks this proportion had increased rather than declined; over a third of patients, at both time points, classified the backaches as severe. Around

70% reported perineal or Caesarean wound pain at 2 weeks and for over a third, this was classified as severe. Nearly half were still experiencing pain at 12 weeks. Over 20% of women reported problems of leaking urine at 2 weeks, and at 12 weeks this proportion had increased, rather than declined, to around 30% (McCourt & Page 1996). Although for the majority the problem was occasional and was classified as mild rather than severe, quite a significant proportion reported impact on everyday activities such as walking and sitting down.

Such problems have the potential to impact negatively on the quality of women's lives and relationships with their babies in the postnatal period. In this study, a significant number of women reported stopping breastfeeding between 2 and 12 weeks post-natally, and reasons given included tiredness, demands of other children, sore or cracked nipples and feeling too tied down (McCourt & Page 1996). Although the great majority of women reported that they enjoyed looking after the baby and felt they were good mothers, over half felt that life was more difficult and that they needed more time to themselves, and over 20% of those who were breastfeeding, at both time points, reported that they did not enjoy it (McCourt & Page 1996). A follow-up study, 5 years later, reported similar levels of morbidity (McCourt & Beake 2001). Over 40% of women felt that the new baby affected the way they got on with their husband or partner, and although the great majority enjoyed looking after the new baby and felt they were good mothers, over half reported finding life much more difficult and over two-thirds felt they needed much more time to themselves (McCourt & Beake 2001).

In a randomised controlled trial (RCT) to test the physical and psychological health effects of a more individualised and long-term model of community-based postnatal care (MacArthur *et al.* 2002, 2003), women in both the intervention and standard care groups completed several validated scales (short form, (SF-36) and the Edinburgh Postnatal Depression Scale (EPDS)) to indicate overall physical and psychological health at 4 and 12 months after the birth, and also reported their experience of postnatal symptoms in the 12-month questionnaire. At 4 months post-natally, 21.25% of women in standard care and 14.39% of women in the intervention care group had EPDS scores of 13 or more, 13 being a level indicating probable depression (Cox & Holden 1994). Additionally, at the 12-month follow-up point, these rates had scarcely declined (although mean scores had decreased, 21.6% and 12.24% still scored 13 or more). A higher proportion of women receiving the new model of care had talked to a midwife about their health problems, and felt it was not difficult to talk to a midwife about them (MacArthur *et al.* 2003). A number of women reported morbidities that were still persisting after 12 months including backache, headache, fatigue (over 20%), stress incontinence (over 15%) and haemorrhoids (over 10%).

Postnatal care and support: the role of midwives

A service led by midwives, with the involvement of women, is at the centre of UK maternity care recommendations (Department of Health 1993, 2004, 2007). According to the UK Department of Health's National Service Framework for Children, Young People and Maternity Services (Department of Health 2004), women need to be provided with a postnatal care service that identifies and responds in a structured and systematic way to their individual physical, psychological, emotional and social needs, and which is based on the best available evidence. The National Institute for Health and Clinical Excellence (NICE) clinical guidelines for postnatal care (NICE 2006a), recommend the provision of personalised care for mothers and babies during the postnatal period, including support for breastfeeding and how to deal with common health problems instead of the currently more common 'tick-box' approach. In addition to providing midwifery care that focuses on the identification and management of women's physical and psychological health after birth, the provision of care should be supportive and sensitive to women's individual needs and preferences. This policy responds to evidence such as MacArthur *et al.*'s RCT of individualised midwifery-led care (described above). This model enabled midwives to design a care package based around structured assessment of each woman's needs and to continue care for a longer time period if required. Their study found significant reductions in postnatal depression symptoms and improvements in certain domains of health for the women receiving this approach, compared with usual postnatal care (MacArthur *et al.* 2002, 2003).

However, even in a country such as the United Kingdom, which has such clear policy support for postnatal care, research indicates that these aims are not being achieved. Many women report experiencing very limited care in hospital, with sometimes insensitive and off-hand care on the part of professionals, and although postnatal home visits are appreciated, community midwives tend to have high caseloads often leading to rushed visits, using a routine and checklist-oriented approach (Garcia *et al.* 1998; Beake *et al.* 2005). The model of care studied by MacArthur *et al.* (2002, 2003) has not been rolled out in practice, except in specific models of care such as caseload practice, where midwives have more autonomy and control over their time to facilitate more individualised approaches to meeting women's and families' needs (McCourt *et al.* 2006a). In such a service context, postnatal morbidity is easily overlooked. In countries, which do not have domiciliary postnatal care, women must take the initiative to seek help for problems, and attend clinics at a time when they are feeling tired and may not always be coping well, so that problems of access to care may arise. In either scenario, there are risks that not only will care lack sensitivity, so that women's feelings may be overlooked, but it may also fail to observe significant physical health problems.

The patterns of postnatal care from midwives differ widely across different countries. In the United Kingdom, home visiting by midwives has been long established, and women expect to receive support at home from midwives, for 10 days, or sometimes for up to 28 days (Department of Health 2004, 2007). This is also followed by an initial home visit by a health visitor, following which women may attend community-based clinics for health checks, immunisations and advice on baby care. This is in contrast to some Western countries, such as the United States, where domiciliary care is not the norm and not universally provided. A number of studies of postnatal support in the United States, therefore, are based on limited schemes targeted towards families or mothers in particular risk categories, and these have varied widely in their effectiveness (Bennett *et al.* 2007). In some European countries the need to further discuss and specify the aims of postnatal care, taking into account the challenge of providing high-quality care after childbirth, is discussed in the light of a development characterised by a continuous reduction in the length of hospital stay, in combination with increasing public demands for information and individualised care (Vendittelli *et al.* 2005; Rudman & Waldenström 2007; Carlgren & Berg 2008).

Similar to the United Kingdom and other high-income countries, length of stay in hospital after birth has declined over the last decade, but levels of home-based postnatal support by professionals have not increased as a result, meaning that hospital-based midwives are providing care for a rapid turnover of women, with little time to get to know their needs or provide support, and community-based midwives have less time available for each postnatal visit. Although 'selective visiting' according to women's needs is encouraged in national policy in the United Kingdom, in practice, the pattern may often depend more on practical considerations than the assessment of each woman's needs and wishes (Beake *et al.* 2005).

Levels and types of informal support – from family, neighbourhoods and friends – also vary in different cultural and social settings as well as for different individuals. Examples from two qualitative studies in the United Kingdom can illustrate this. The first involved interviews with a diverse sample of women who had given birth in a London teaching hospital, using a narrative approach to recount their maternity experience and views (Beake *et al.* 2005). The women in this study, and in the wider survey of which they formed a sample (McCourt & Beake 2001), were more critical of postnatal care in hospital than in any other aspect of care. They felt that their ordinary needs for practical, emotional and informational support were not being met and some women spoke of feeling abandoned on the postnatal wards:

> I kept asking for help with feeding but nobody would come and if they did it was like about a minute and then the next day somebody said 'do you want to go home'.

The quality of the support received was also a matter of concern, as some women also reported feeling undermined by midwives' responses to their needs for help. In hospital, women are particularly dependent on professional support as they are in the early stage of recovering from the birth, and they are relatively isolated from the informal support that their partners, family and friends might provide. Additionally, women may lack experience of new babies and need information and reassurance as well as practical help. This woman, for example, was upset by a midwife's response to her request for help for what clearly, to the midwife, seemed a trivial issue:

> so (first baby) had all this black stuff that comes out after the baby comes into the world, like pooh, but it is so horrid and I was terrified because it was so much... I rang the bell, it was 3 o' clock. I said 'look at this'. She said 'so, (shouting tone) she was expecting to have this, are you calling me just for this, just change the nappy and go back to bed' and walked out of the room.

It is easy for midwives to forget that what seems routine and unimportant to them may feel very different for a mother struggling to adjust to caring for a new baby while also recovering from giving birth. In contrast, those women who felt they had been given support appreciated this greatly. The woman quoted below felt she had a lot of help following her Caesarean birth, including taking the baby at night when crying so that she could rest. She was also more positive about the midwives' attitudes:

> having 24 hour a day somebody who knows what they are talking about and can talk to you in a way that you can understand and appreciate. None of them ever lost their cool or anything, even though you could see they were busy.

The women's views of postnatal care at home were more positive and they appreciated the availability of midwives to visit at home, but they often found the care to be routine and rushed, with the result that more time-consuming issues such as breastfeeding problems or feelings of low mood and difficulty in coping could not be attended to sufficiently (Beake *et al.* 2005).

The second study we refer to involved interviews, using a similar approach, with a sample of women in a neighbourhood with a high proportion of South Asian women and other minority ethnic groups (McCourt *et al.* 2006b). The majority of the respondents were South Asian women of Indian origin. These women held very similar views of hospital postnatal care, for example:

After the birth I did not have any help at all until I came home.

One midwife (from the community group practice) came to check the baby. She did remove the stitches and done everything. The hospital people, some really don't know what they are doing. There is no communication with each other. They are not doing a good service, they don't really care enough about people.

Most lived within extended families or had relatives living nearby and reported that they had plenty of practical support at home. They did not have the same reliance on professionals for practical or emotional support, and those who were not born in the United Kingdom explained that such professional support would not have been available in their home country. Nonetheless, they felt strongly that such support should be available, as professionals cannot assume that women have good informal support, and because they have particular expertise and information to offer, for example, in dealing with breastfeeding problems:

The midwife tells us to do it in a certain way and she will say 'if you do it that way you get back pain' so it's things like that which is helpful. Even our parents don't know all about this.

From the above discussion, it is clear that even women who have a healthy pregnancy and straightforward birth commonly experience a number of difficult postnatal symptoms and may find the challenges of caring for a new baby exhausting and difficult, as well as rewarding and joyful. For an increasing proportion of women, worldwide, they commence their new lives with their baby following a difficult or even traumatic birth, or in difficult social circumstances and many lack good sources of ordinary support, increasing their reliance on professionals to cope with the early days of recovery and adjustment (McCourt 2006). The evidence from women's views suggests that their post-partum physical, emotional and psychological health needs are not being fully addressed by current practice, which tends to include routine observations and examinations that are often unnecessary (MacArthur *et al.* 2003). Studies describing women's experience of staff attitudes in early postnatal care show that often women felt poorly prepared for the postnatal period, needed more information about their own health and complained of the lack of support, and that they were also critical about the inconsistency of advice and the lack of evidence-based and realistic information (Beake *et al.* 2005).

This suggests that midwifery care is very much a balancing act. It is important for midwives to not only be able to recognise morbidity and respond appropriately, giving enough care and support, and referring for medical care when appropriate, but also to avoid pathologising common postnatal problems, and encourage women to use their own, informal sources of support. Midwives also need to reassure women by letting them know that some health problems and difficulties are 'normal' in the sense of being frequently experienced after childbirth, and supporting them where possible to take up ordinary sources of support, such as, help from friends, neighbours and family so that they can rest and recover. In the following sections we look in more depth at three aspects of postnatal care that studies have shown to be important, but often overlooked in practice: perineal care, post Caesarean care and support for women with mental health problems such as post-traumatic stress following childbirth.

Care of the perineum

Childbirth is a genital experience and, if not managed accordingly, can bring enduring postnatal morbidity that can affect women's physical, psychological and social health. Some factors during a vaginal birth can be modified in attempts to preserve as much functional integrity to the perineum as possible. Skilful care of the perineum during birth and the puerperium is one of the major contributions that midwives can make to the comfort and well-being of childbearing women. The midwife is the most skilled healthcare professional assisting women during the majority of normal births in many countries and has the responsibility of deciding how to manage the perineum and whether or not to perform an episiotomy, as well as the responsibility for the repair of perineal trauma. Episiotomy and perineal trauma result in unnecessary pain and may lead to longer term problems, such as painful intercourse. All in all, perineal management and care falls under the remit of the midwife's sphere of responsibility.

Perineal care has traditionally been a key, routine component of post-natal checks, in hospital and home-based care. However, it is not clear despite this, if midwives and other healthcare professionals give sufficient attention to this aspect of care, despite its potential impact on women's well-being and quality of life (Bick & MacArthur 1994). Additionally, recent changes in care, in order to avoid routine practices, may have discouraged midwives from proactively checking women's perineal healing, relying instead on women to report problems

(Bick & MacArthur 1994, 1995). In the context of rushed visits, however, women may not always feel able to raise concerns and ask questions (McCourt 2006). Additionally, women, often experiencing perineal trauma for the first time and with little information available publicly, may not feel confident in knowing what is normal healing and recovery.

Even with a clear focus on recovery following childbirth, important adverse long-term health effects of perineal trauma that are likely to have an impact on the well-being of women may be overlooked. These include perineal pain, painful sexual intercourse, altered urinary function and anal incontinence (Eason *et al.* 2002), all of which are correlated with obstetric intervention but can also occur after normal birth (MacArthur *et al.* 1991, 1997, 2001; Johanson *et al.* 1993; Glazener *et al.* 1995; Glazener 1997; Sultan *et al.* 1997; Signorello *et al.* 2001; Van Kessel *et al.* 2001; Williams *et al.* 2007). Because such problems may remain hidden, health-care professionals need to ask women if they have any problems and if they have any fears or worries. If such issues are not addressed, there is the potential for long-term problems as a result of trauma, including both physical symptoms and psychological issues such as possible fears of further pregnancy and birth (Gamble & Creedy 2005). There is some evidence that maternal requests for elective Caesarean section are primarily motivated by such fears (Weaver *et al.* 2001; McCourt *et al.* 2007; Weaver 2007). Although the numbers of women involved in exploring this issue are small, this may potentially grow, leading to further health problems in future, and therefore, the issue of women's fears of birth is now being reflected in development of consultant midwives' clinics to tackle such concerns in subsequent pregnancies (Dunkley-Bent 2004).

Studies examining specific factors in women's post-partum health such as perineal trauma and pain have found that the more severe the perineal trauma the greater the incidence of perineal pain at days 1 and 7 following the birth (Macarthur & Macarthur 2004). In the 'Hands On Or Poised' (HOOP) trial of perineal care, McCandlish *et al.* (1998) found that 85% of women experienced some form of perineal trauma (Albers *et al.* 1999b). Perineal pain with one or more daily activities, such as walking, sitting, breastfeeding, bowel movements or urination and sexual intercourse are commonly reported symptoms following vaginal birth (Thompson *et al.* 2000). These problems are especially relevant to women having their first baby and to women who had had an episiotomy and/or instrumental birth (Thompson 2002). Research also indicates that women report more pain if they had perineal trauma with suturing (Albers *et al.* 1999a). It is evident from these studies that recovery following childbirth can be longer than anticipated and have serious implications on a woman's reproductive and sexual life and affect more women than midwives and health professionals may have previously thought.

Urinary and also anal incontinence, represents a major source of personal and social embarrassment, which can undermine the quality of life of many women. Any measure that can treat the condition at an early stage will enhance women's confidence. Childbirth may induce either mechanical or neurologic injury to the pelvic floor muscles and anal sphincter. Weakness of these muscles caused by stretching during pregnancy and delivery has been a possible explanation for post-partum urinary incontinence (Snooks *et al.* 1984). The NICE recommendations for incontinence in women state that 'Most women with post-partum incontinence should be managed conservatively' (NICE 2006b). Research suggests that anal and urinary incontinence following vaginal birth may result from damage to the innervations of the pelvic floor muscles, rather than the stretching of muscles, and for some women there is uncertainty if pelvic floor exercises alone may have any value in preventing incontinence (Glazener *et al.* 2005).

The complexity of genital tract trauma sustained in childbirth has a direct relationship with subsequent pain and functional impairment (Albers *et al.* 1999a; Macarthur & Macarthur 2004). While giving birth over an intact perineum may require additional time in the second stage of labour and greater patience from the birth attendant, it is associated with fewer maternal health problems in the short run (blood loss, pain, and need for suturing) and in the long run (continued pain, pelvic floor weakness, sexual problems, and bowel and urinary incontinence) (Albers & Borders 2007). Much remains to be learned about minimising genital tract trauma in vaginal birth, and strategies that acknowledge labour and birth as a normal physiologic event, avoiding interventions for women without complications, are elements of care most likely to promote women's health and comfort and cause no harm, which are the hallmarks of midwifery practice.

Studies such as the ones described in this chapter have important implications for midwifery practice and education. Midwives should focus on providing evidence-based practice and advice, and not base their care simply on tradition or personal preference; only this way will women receive care most likely to be effective and beneficial. Similarly, healthcare providers must foster support for the implementation of research findings into practice, facilitating and encouraging a multidisciplinary team approach committed to improving the quality of perineal management during birth and providing care that is sensitive to women's needs in the post-partum period. All aspects of perineal management and care are challenging for midwives and healthcare services providing maternity care. Women trust professionals' judgement and we must ensure that the care we are providing does not misplace this trust.

Postnatal care following Caesarean birth

As we have noted, operative birth is becoming increasingly common; therefore, a significant proportion of women in the postnatal period are recovering from major or minor surgery (such as forceps birth and episiotomy) as well as learning to care for their baby, and adjusting to the enormous life changes they are experiencing (McCourt 2006). The World Health Organisation (WHO) recommends a rate of Caesarean section of around 10–15% to protect maternal and infant well-being, but the rates in many countries are far in excess of these. In resource-rich 'Western' countries such as the United Kingdom, rates have reached around 20–30% (which is double the WHO level, Villar *et al.* 2006) and rises are increasingly being found in middle-income and less industrialised countries. In countries with privatised healthcare systems or medically led maternity services, rates may be even higher (Murray 2000). Additionally, an 'inverse care law' has been highlighted, where poor and rural women often experience rates far below the recommended level, while richer and urban women in the same countries may experience rates far in excess of this (DeClercq 2008).

One consequence of such rising rates is that this major abdominal operation is coming to be treated in a more routine manner. Language used in the media and by some obstetricians illustrates this issue well, with the operation being described in terms such as a 'nice clean cut' (Fisk 1997). The potential risks, and the consequences for postnatal morbidity (Lilford *et al.* 1990) are given relatively limited attention, to the degree where media headlines can describe women having elective Caesarean sections as 'too posh to push' (Weaver 2007) with little regard for the problems, which may lead to elective operations (McCourt *et al.* 2007; Weaver 2007), or the problems, such as severe pain, that the women may experience post-natally. Caesarean section has been shown to have a major impact on women's health and quality of life post-natally (Lydon-Rochelle *et al.* 2000; Lavender *et al.* 2006; Villar *et al.* 2007) in the short term, and major long-term impact in relation to future pregnancies and births (Smith *et al.* 2003; Ash *et al.* 2007). Long-term consequences include the need for repeat Caesarean section, which in itself becomes more risky with each subsequent delivery and placental problems (Amu *et al.* 1998; Bewley & Cockburn 2002). However, the main focus of postnatal care is the short-term consequences, which may be both physical and psychological. Common physical problems include scar pain and wound infection, and a woman, following Caesarean, may be much more likely to have an infected uterus than a woman who had a vaginal birth. A woman who had a Caesarean appears to be more likely than a woman who had a vaginal birth to have blood clots, including pulmonary embolism and stroke. Apart from having a wound that needs post-operative monitoring and care, a woman who had a Caesarean may also be injured from accidental cuts to nearby organs such as the bladder or bowel or urethra.

In the United Kingdom, as Caesarean birth rates have increased, the length of women's hospital stay following the operation has fallen. In 1995, the typical length of hospital stay following Caesarean birth was around 7 days (McCourt & Page 1996; McCourt & Beake 2001); by 2005, this had fallen to about 3 or 4 days (Department of Health 2005). Additionally, there is evidence that during their hospital stay, women recovering from Caesarean birth may receive very limited care owing to staff shortages and busyness (Beake *et al.* 2005). The following quotes, from a study of women's experiences of birth (McCourt & Page 1996), illustrate that feeling abandoned and lacking in practical help following birth was not confined to healthy women who had experienced normal birth:

> well, the care on the wards was not, while they are good on the labour ward they are not the most polite people in the world. I hate to say they do want to hurry you out, definitely . . . it is as if after the birth, you are a burden to them, hurry up and get out. They give you no support whatsoever, although this time around they were slightly better because my baby was in intensive care, so I did have a reason to be in hospital.

Another woman had suffered domestic violence in pregnancy, and felt she needed, but did not receive, a lot of moral support in pregnancy. Following her Caesarean birth, while day staff were helpful she found the night staff much less so and this had an impact on her ability to cope:

> (baby) decided he wanted to go to the toilet and have something to eat at the same time . . . so I changed him while he was on the bed, but he was screaming the place down and she came into me and said 'feed your baby' and I went mad. I went mad because I had no sleep, I'm still trying to recover from the Caesarean, I've got no experience whatsoever with the baby. This is only the second night, I don't know, he's making me sleep, I'm tired, I want to go to sleep. All I want him to do is shut up and he is crying and she is telling me about feeding the baby. . .

The impact on psychological well-being is equally important, and may affect women in different ways according to whether their operation was a planned or emergency intervention, and also influenced by the quality of care and support they received. There is evidence, for example, that women who felt well informed and that they had some measure of control over events fared better psychologically than those who did not (Green & Baston 2003).

DiMatteo *et al.* (1996) meta-analysis of psychosocial outcomes following Caesarean delivery reviewed 43 quantitative studies and found generally worse psychological outcomes for planned and intrapartum Caesarean compared with vaginal birth, including general satisfaction, rates of breastfeeding and how positively they evaluated their babies. The experience also had a negative impact on subsequent childbearing. Barnes *et al.*'s (2007) study of negative emotions following childbirth found a significant association between Caesarean birth and negative feelings, including the use of more negative words to describe the baby. Other studies have found associations between Caesarean birth and delays in future childbearing or decisions not to become pregnant (Porter *et al.* 2006). Consequently, women who have experienced Caesarean delivery need higher levels of postnatal support, attending to both their physical and psychological needs.

In a study of women's views on the impact of operative delivery (including Caesarean section) in the second stage of labour, Murphy *et al.* (2003) found that the majority of women did not feel they had sufficient 'debriefing' or explanation of the reasons. Some felt that the emotional impact of operative delivery had not been addressed and a number of them described anxieties around future births sufficient to deter them from becoming pregnant again. Similarly, in Robb's (2007) phenomenological study of Canadian women's experiences of intrapartum Caesarean section, the women described 'a cascade of immediate and lingering emotional reactions' including disappointment, sadness, inadequacy and fear (Robb 2007: 3). Their reactions, however, could be mediated by aspects of care, particularly the quality of support given by a midwife, information provision and whether they felt in control (Robb 2007). The women also advocated being given the opportunity for an obstetric review at about 3 months following birth.

Postnatal mental health and post-traumatic stress

As we have discussed, psychological problems post-natally may be as common as physical symptoms, and maternal postnatal mental health has an important impact on the well-being of the woman, her infant and her family. Postnatal psychological morbidity can be associated with a range of factors including earlier life experiences and mental health problems, poor levels of postnatal support and traumatic birth experiences (Robertson *et al.* 2004; Leigh & Milgrom 2008). Therefore, at each postnatal contact, women should be asked about their emotional well-being, what family and social support they have and their usual coping strategies for dealing with everyday matters. Women and their families/partners should be encouraged to tell their healthcare professional about any changes in mood, emotional state and behaviour that are outside of the woman's normal pattern (NICE 2007).

Healthcare professionals should be alert to women's mental health problems in the postnatal period, including the onset of new disorders such as postnatal depression (PND), puerperal psychosis, post-traumatic stress disorder and panic disorder and relapse of other psychotic illnesses, such as schizophrenia. Women with existing diagnoses should be identified during admission and care plans for postnatal management adhered to, based on their current mental state and risk of relapse (NICE 2007).

We have noted that depression following childbirth is common, well known and has been widely researched and debated. Postnatal post-traumatic stress disorder (PN PTSD) or 'birth trauma' (Beck 2004), which refers to a disorder that can occur in women following the experience or witnessing of life-threatening events in childbirth has increasingly attracted the attention of public health researchers, but is less widely known among health professionals providing postnatal care. In the United Kingdom, an estimated 6–10% of women present with clinical symptoms of PTSD following childbirth. When PN PTSD develops, its symptoms may start soon after childbirth or be delayed for months. The symptoms may persist for a long time and result in other problems such as PND, although the two disorders have different origins. Both require early diagnosis, specialised care and treatment. General symptoms of PTSD include the following (Diagnostic and Statistical Manual of the American Psychiatric Association 1994):

- Persistent re-experiencing of the event by way of recurrent intrusive memories, flashbacks and nightmares
- Avoidance of anything that reminds them of the trauma, which can lead to emotional detachment or numbing
- 'Hyperarousal' symptoms – irritability, difficulties with sleeping and concentrating

Women can feel traumatised by labour regardless of the mode of birth. However, invasive obstetric procedures such as emergency Caesarean sections, labour inductions and instrumental vaginal births are more likely to be perceived as traumatic and are associated with PTSD. postnatal debriefing for at-risk women has been suggested as a way of preventing both PTSD and PND, although evidence of its effectiveness is lacking (Rowan *et al.* 2007). The term *debriefing* has been much discussed in recent midwifery literature, but is poorly understood and is often used by midwives interchangeably with other concepts such as postnatal review, counselling or support. Additionally, each approach requires more research to assess effectiveness. Psychological debriefing is an intervention that was developed with the aim of helping people to cope with a traumatic event, initially used in situations such as war and disaster, and later extended to other forms of trauma. Rose and Tehrani (2002, p. 3) describe the psychological model as generally involving 'a slow sequential exposition of the event' with the aim of achieving cognitive restructuring while recognising grief. The principle is to revisit and recount emotional responses and sensory experiences during the event as well as retelling of the facts of it, with the idea that a 'ventilation' of emotional responses will be therapeutic.

Rose and Tehrani (2002) note that, while such an approach was widely assumed to be beneficial, this has been debated, and research on effectiveness has confirmed questions about the approach. Such complex subjects and interventions are difficult to research, particularly where interventions studied may vary in quality and approach, and may be applied to different kinds of trauma (Ormerod 2002). However, it has been suggested that early interventions of this type may be superimposed on or may even interfere with a natural recovery process, may medicalise normal distress or replace individuals' own means of coping with traumatic experiences, or even that the arousal at this early stage may serve to re-traumatise the individual (Ormerod 2002). The recommendation of NICE guidelines, consequently, is that debriefing should not be routinely offered, or offered within a month of a traumatic experience. After 1 month, those individuals who may be vulnerable to PTSD can be identified at this stage and offered appropriate review, counselling or debriefing (Department of Health 2001; NICE 2007).

The psychological debriefing approach is not necessarily equivalent to review or counselling by midwives or obstetricians following a traumatic birth, but with limited research available on maternity care, the advice regarding timing of review should be followed. The recommended timing also relates well to the woman's need for a period of rest and recovery following childbirth. This also indicates the potentially long-term nature of the need for postnatal support, and value of a model of postnatal care that can allow midwives to assess women's individual needs and continue care for a month if required (MacArthur *et al.* 2002). Two of the studies included in the Cochrane Review of debriefing were focused on maternity care (Lavender & Walkinshaw 1998; Small *et al.* 2000) and the reviewers noted that the approaches in these studies were somewhat different, in being more 'patient-led' and delivered by midwives, so may not have shared the full characteristics of a 'psychological debriefing' approach. Additionally, neither study looked at PTSD symptoms per se. Clearly, further research is needed on the subject of postnatal interventions relating to birth traumas, but midwives should be aware that a number of women may suffer damaging symptoms of PTSD, in addition to those who suffer from better-known problems such as depression, should therefore be asking women about their emotional health following childbirth and be equipped to offer advice or referral if needed. Gamble and Creedy (2004), in a review of counselling-type interventions after distressing birth experiences, note that further research is needed to investigate different types of counselling and their effects, and also, that interventions are provided in a context of inadequate postnatal support for most women, including limited opportunities for midwives to listen to women talk about their birth experiences and how they are feeling.

Conclusion

This chapter has discussed the types of morbidity that women commonly experience after childbirth, including physical and psychological problems. We have noted that the rates of symptoms of morbidity are high and that problems are often under-reported as women may feel embarrassed or that they should not 'bother' health professionals with minor problems. However, even relatively minor problems may have an important impact on the quality of a woman's life and her ability to care for and enjoy the time with her new baby. Maternal mental health problems have been shown to have a major impact on the development of infants, and a negative impact is not confined to those with the more major and acute psychological morbidities such as puerperal psychosis (Beck 1995).

Within this context, midwives face the challenge to strike a good balance in offering care and support to women – to provide reassurance and take a positive approach, and also to take the potential impact of postnatal morbidity seriously and offer adequate care, referring women for more specialist care when needed.

Reassuring women that some of the longer term morbidity following childbirth may be difficult to treat and that it might not resolve completely but in general be alleviated with information, discussion, support and reassurance from a knowledgeable individual could result in women feeling better about themselves.

We have also discussed the variability and changes in the ways in which postnatal care is provided. In many countries, domiciliary postnatal care is not provided routinely, leaving the onus on women to visit healthcare facilities if they experience problems. While routine services are not always beneficial, the considerable evidence of under-reporting of postnatal morbidity and its potentially negative impact on women's quality of life and well-being suggests that there are particular advantages to providing domiciliary care. The importance of this is likely to have increased in the United Kingdom and in many other countries where lengths of hospital stay post-natally have declined considerably in the recent past. Additionally, studies of women's views of maternity care show that women value postnatal care at home highly and are generally more satisfied with this than with the care in hospital (Dowswell *et al.* 2001). In a situation where time and resources for care are limited, the most optimal care is likely to be provided by flexibly offering care around women's and families' needs, such as the model of care assessed in MacArthur and Bick's trial of woman-centred care packages. Some women are able to cope well after birth, suffer few health problems or are able to draw on their own sources of informal support, and therefore may not need frequent or intensive postnatal care by midwives, while others will need and benefit from greater support from midwives. Taking a woman-centred approach will support midwives in being able to provide appropriate forms and levels of care.

Key implications for midwifery practice

- It is very common for women to experience a number of postnatal health problems. Most commonly reported physical morbidities are back pain, urinary or faecal incontinence, perineal pain, intercourse problems, breast problems, haemorrhoids, constipation and headaches.
- Although women may need reassurance that many health problems are common, they should be offered adequate care and attention to these problems and their impact on women's and families' lives acknowledged.
- Women often do not report their symptoms, so midwives need to be observant and proactive in asking about each woman's well-being and responding to problems.
- Although the value of routine physical checks has been questioned, midwives cannot assume that women will report all problems, and sufficient attention should be given to perineal care and healing.
- Psychological problems are also common after birth and may have a major impact on the future well-being of the woman and her family. Midwives should ask women about their mental health as well as their physical well-being, and be aware of appropriate forms of support and referral.
- A more women and family-centred approach to postnatal care is needed.

Points for reflection on your practice:

In providing postnatal care, how far are you able to give women the level and type of care that they need?

What influences this?

In community settings, do you conduct selective visits, and if so, how far is the pattern of visiting based on assessment of the individual woman and family's needs?

References

Abraham A (2004) Lack of communication affects the care of patients and families. *Professional Nurse* Feb, 19 (6): 351–353 (accessed 22/07/2009).

Albers LL, Borders N (2007) Minimizing genital tract trauma and related pain following spontaneous vaginal birth. *Journal of Midwifery and Women's Health* 52 (3): 246–253.

Albers LL, Garcia J, Renfrew M, McCandlish R, Elbourne D (1999a) Distribution of genital tract trauma in childbirth and related postnatal pain. *Birth* 26 (1): 11–17.

Albers LL, Sedler KD, Greulich B (1999b) In the literature: midwifery care: the "gold standard" for normal childbirth? *Birth* 26 (1): 53–54.

Amu O, Rajendran S, Bolaji II (1998) Controversies in management: should doctors perform an elective Caesarean section on request? Maternal choice alone should not determine method of delivery. *British Medical Journal* 317: 463–465.

Ash A, Smith A, Maxwell D (2007) Caesarean scar pregnancy. *British Journal of Obstetrics and Gynaecology* 114 (3): 253–263.

Barclay L, Everitt L, Rogan F, Schmied V, Wyllie A (1997) Becoming a mother – an analysis of women's experience of early motherhood. *Journal of Advanced Nursing* 25: 719–728.

Barnes J, Ram B, Leach P, *et al.* (2007) Factors associated with negative emotional expression: a study of mothers of young infants. Families, Children and Child Care Project (FCCC) Team. *Journal of Reproductive and Infant Psychology* 25 (2): 122–138.

Beake S, McCourt C, Bick DE (2005) Women's views of hospital and community-based postnatal care: the good, the bad and the indifferent. *Evidence-Based Midwifery* 3 (2): 80–86.

Beck CT (1995) The effects of postpartum depression on maternal–infant interaction: a meta-analysis. *Nursing Research* 44 (5): 298–304.

Beck CT (2002) Postpartum depression: a metasynthesis. *Quality and Health Research* 12: 453–472.

Beck CT (2004) Birth trauma: in the eye of the beholder. *Nursing Research* 53 (1): 28–35.

Bennett C, Macdonald GM, Dennis J, *et al.* (2007) Home-based support for disadvantaged adult mothers. *Cochrane Database of Systematic Reviews* (3).

Bewley S, Cockburn J (2002) The unethics of 'request' caesarean section. *British Journal of Obstetrics and Gynaecology* 109: 593–596.

Bick D, MacArthur C (1994) Identifying morbidity in postpartum women. *Modern Midwife* 4 (12): 10–13.

Bick DE, MacArthur C (1995) The extent, severity and effect of health problems after childbirth. *British Journal of Midwifery* 3 (27): 31.

Brown S, Lumley J (1998) Maternal health after childbirth: results of an Australian population-based survey. *British Journal of Obstetrics and Gynaecology* 105: 156–161.

Brown S, Lumley J (2000) Physical health problems after childbirth and maternal depression at six to seven months postpartum. *British Journal of Obstetrics and Gynaecology* 107 (10): 1194–1201.

Carlgren I, Berg M (2008) Postpartum consultation: occurrence, requirements and expectations. *BMC Pregnancy and Childbirth* 8: 29.

Cox J, Holden J (eds) (1994) *Perinatal Psychiatry. Use and Misuse of the Edinburgh Postnatal Depression Scale*. London: Gaskell (Royal College of Psychiatrists).

DeClercq E (2008) Cesarean birth in the United States: epidemiology, trends, and outcomes. Presentation at the International Confederation of Midwives Triennial Conference (ICM Conference), Glasgow, Scotland, June 2008.

Department of Health (1993) *Changing Childbirth, Report of the Expert Maternity Group*. London: HMSO.

Department of Health (2001) *Treatment Choice in Psychological Therapies and Counselling–Evidence-based Clinical Practice Guidelines*. London: HMSO.

Department of Health (2004) *National Services Framework for Children, Young people and Maternity Services*. London: The Stationery Office.

Department of Health (2005) *NHS Maternity Statistics, England: 2003-4 Bulletin 2005/10*. London: Department of Health.

Department of Health (2007) *Maternity Matters: Choice, Access and Continuity of Care in a Safe Service*. London: The Stationery Office.

DiMatteo MR, Morton SC, Lepper HS, *et al.* (1996) Cesarean childbirth and psychosocial outcomes: a meta-analysis. *Health Psychology* 15 (4): 303–314.

Dowswell T, Renfrew MJ, Gregson B, Hewison J (2001) A review of the literature on women's views on their maternity care in the community in the UK. *Midwifery* Sep, 17 (3): 194–202.

Dunkley-Bent J (2004) A consultant midwife's community clinic. *British Journal of Midwifery* 12 (3): 144–171.

Eason E, Labrecque M, Marcoux S, Mondor M (2002) Anal incontinence after childbirth. *CMAJ: Canadian Medical Association Journal* 166 (3): 326–330.

Fisk N (1997) The benefits of having a nice, clean cut. Interview by Sue Corrigan. *The Times*, Tuesday, July 15, 1997.

Gamble J, Creedy D (2004) Content and processes of postpartum counseling after a distressing birth experience: a review. *Birth* 31 (3): 213–218.

Gamble J, Creedy D (2005) Psychological trauma symptoms of operative birth. *British Journal of Midwifery* 13 (4): 218–224.

Garcia J, Redshaw M, Fitzsimmons B, Keene J (1998) *First Class Delivery: A National Survey of Woman's Views on Maternity Care*. London: Audit Commission.

Glazener CM (1997) Sexual function after childbirth; women's experiences, persistent morbidity and lack of professional recognition. *British Journal of Obstetrics and Gynaecology* 104: 330–335.

Glazener C, Abdalla M, Stroud S, Naji S, Templeton A, Russell I (1995) Postnatal maternal morbidity: extent, causes, prevention and treatment. *British Journal of Obstetrics and Gynaecology* 102: 282–287.

Glazener CM, Herbison GP, MacArthur C, Grant A, Wilson PD (2005) Randomised controlled trial of conservative management of postnatal urinary and faecal incontinence: six year follow up. *British Medical Journal* 330 (7487): 337.

Green J, Baston H (2003) Feeling in control during labor: concepts, correlates, and consequences. *Birth* 30 (4): 235–247.

Hodnett E, Fredericks S (2007) Support during pregnancy for women at increased risk of low birthweight babies (review). *The Cochrane Library* (4).

Johanson R, Wilkinson P, Bastible A, Ryan S, Murphy H, O'Brien S (1993) Health after childbirth: a comparison of normal and assisted vaginal delivery. *Midwifery* 9 (3): 161–168.

Jordan B (1993) Birth in four cultures. *A Crosscultural Investigation of Childbirth in Yucatan, Holland, Sweden and the United States.* Illinois: Waveland Press.

Lavender T, Hofmeyr GJ, Neilson JP, Kingdon C, Gyte GML (2006) Caesarean Section for Non-medical Reasons at Term. *Cochrane Database of Systematic Reviews* 3. Art. No.: CD004660.

Lavender T, Walkinshaw SA (1998) Can midwives reduce postpartum psychological morbidity? A randomised controlled trial. *Birth* 25 (4): 215–219.

Leigh B, Milgrom J (2008) Risk factors for antenatal depression, postnatal depression and parenting stress. *BMC Psychiatry* 8: 24.

Lewis G (ed.) (2004) *Why Mothers Die. Confidential Enquiry into Maternal and Child Health.* London: RCOG.

Lewis G (ed.) The Confidential Enquiry into Maternal and Child Health (CEMACH) (2007) Saving Mothers' Lives. *The Seventh Report on Confidential Enquiries into Maternal Deaths in the United Kingdom.* London: The Stationery Office.

Lilford RJ, van Coeverden de Groot HA, Moore PJ, Bingham P (1990) The relative risks of caesarean section (intrapartum and elective) and vaginal delivery: a detailed analysis to exclude the effects of medical disorders and other acute pre-existing physiological disturbances. *British Journal of Obstetrics and Gynaecology* 97: 883–892.

Lydon-Rochelle M, Holt V, Martin D, Easterling T (2000) Association between method of delivery and maternal re-hospitalization. *The Journal of the American Medical Association* 283: 2411–2416.

MacArthur C, Bick DE, Keighley MRB (1997) Faecal incontinence after childbirth. *British Journal of Obstetrics and Gynaecology* 104: 46–50.

MacArthur C, Glazener CM, Wilson PD, Herbison GP, Gee H, Lang GD, Lancashire R (2001) Obstetric practice and faecal incontinence three months after delivery. *British Journal of Obstetrics and Gynaecology* Jul, 108 (7): 678–683.

MacArthur C, Lewis M, Knox EG (1991) *Health After Childbirth: An Investigation of Long Term Health Problems Beginning After Childbirth in 11,701 Women.* London: HM Stationery Office.

Macarthur AJ, Macarthur C (2004) Incidence, severity, and determinants of perineal pain after vaginal delivery: a prospective cohort study. *American Journal of Obstetrics and Gynecology* 191 (4): 1199–1204.

MacArthur C, Winter HR, Bick DE, *et al.* (2002) The effects of re-designed community postnatal care on women's health four months after birth: a cluster randomised controlled trial. *The Lancet* 359: 378–385.

MacArthur C, Winter HR, Bick DE, *et al.* (2003) Re-designing postnatal care: a randomised controlled trial of protocol-based midwifery-led care focused on individual women's physical and psychological health needs. *Health Technology Assessment* 7 (37).

Mander R (2001) *Supportive Care and Midwifery*. Oxford: Blackwell.

Maternity Care Working Party (2008) *Making Normal Birth a Reality. Consensus Statement from the Maternity Care Working Party; our Shared Views about the Need to Recognise, Facilitate and Audit Normal Birth*. London: NCT/RCM/RCOG, November 2007.

McCandlish R, Bowler U, van Asten H, *et al.* (1998) A randomised controlled trial of care of the perineum during second stage of normal labour. *British Journal of Obstetrics and Gynaecology* 105 (12): 1262–1272.

McCourt C (2006) Becoming a Parent. In: Page L, McCandlish R (eds). *The New Midwifery. Science and Sensitivity in Practice*. Edinburgh: Churchill Livingstone.

McCourt C (2009) Social Support. In: Squire C (ed.) *The Social Context of Childbirth*, 2nd Edition. Oxford: Radcliffe.

McCourt C, Beake S (2001) Using Midwifery Monitor to assess quality in two maternity care systems. *Practising Midwife* Feb, 4 (2): 23–29.

McCourt C, Beake S, Weaver J, Gamble J, Creedy D (2007) Elective caesarean section and decision making. A critical review of the literature. *Birth* 34: 65–79.

McCourt C, Jetha C, Beake S, McAree T, Stewart S (2006b) *Report on the Evaluation of a Midwifery Group Practice: Perceptions of Consumers and Providers Centre for Research in Midwifery and Childbirth*. London: Thames Valley University.

McCourt C, Page L (1996) *Report on the Evaluation of One-to-One Midwifery*. London: Centre for Midwifery Practice, Thames Valley University, Hammersmith Hospitals NHS Trust. www.health.tvu.ac.uk/mid.

McCourt C, Stevens T, Sandall J, Brodie P (2006a) Working with women: continuity of carer in practice. In: Page L, McCandlish R (eds) *The New Midwifery: Science and Sensitivity in Practice*, 2nd Edition. Oxford: Churchill Livingstone.

Miller T (2002) Adapting to motherhood: care in the postnatal period. *Community Practitioner* 75 (1): 16–18.

Murphy D, Pope C, Frost J, Liebling RE (2003) Qualitative interview study: delivery in the second stage of labour. *British Medical Journal* 327: 1132, doi:10.1136/bmj.327.7424.1132.

Murray S (2000) Qualitative and quantitative study: high rates of caesarean section in Chile. *British Medical Journal* 321: 1501–1505.

National Institute for Health and Clinical Excellence (2006a) *NICE Clinical Guideline 37. Routine Postnatal Care of Women and their Babies*. www.nice.org.uk/CG037fullguideline (accessed 7/2006).

National Institute for Health and Clinical Excellence (2006b) *NICE Clinical Guideline 40. Urinary Incontinence. The Management of Urinary Incontinence in Women*. http://www.nice.org.uk/nicemedia/pdf/CG40NICEguideline.pdf (accessed 10/2006).

National Institute for Health and Clinical Excellence (2007) *NICE Clinical Guideline 45. Antenatal and Postnatal Mental Health: Clinical Management and Service Guidance.* http://www.nice.org.uk/guidance/CG45fullguideline.

Ormerod J (2002) Current research into the effectiveness of debriefing. *Psychological Debriefing*. Leicester: British Psychological Society, Professional Practice Board Working Party. www.bps.org.uk.

Porter M, Bhattacharya S, van Teijlingen E (2006) Unfulfilled expectations: how circumstances impinge on women's reproductive choices. *Social Science and Medicine* 62 (7): 1757–1767.

Robb K (2007) A Phenomenological Study Exploring Women's Experiences of Intrapartum Cesarean Delivery with Midwife or Obstetrician Care in Nova Scotia. MA dissertation, Thames Valley University, London.

Robertson E, Grace S, Wallington T, *et al.* (2004) Antenatal risk factors for postpartum depression: a synthesis of recent literature. *General Hospital Psychiatry* 26: 289–295.

Rose S, Bisson J, Churchill R, Wessely, S, Cochrane Depression, Anxiety and Neurosis Group (2008) Psychological debriefing for preventing post traumatic stress disorder (PTSD) [Systematic Review]. *Cochrane Database of Systematic Reviews* 3.

Rose S, Tehrani N (2002) History, methods and development of psychological debriefing. *Psychological Debriefing*. Leicester: British Psychological Society, Professional Practice Board Working Party. www.bps.org.uk.

Rowan C, Bick D, Bastos MH (2007) Postnatal debriefing interventions to prevent maternal mental health problems after birth: exploring the gap between the evidence and UK policy and practice. *Worldviews in Evidence Based Nursing* 4 (2): 97–105.

Rudman A, Waldenström U (2007) Critical views on postpartum care expressed by new mothers. *BMC Health Services Research* 7: 178.

Signorello LB, Harlow BL, Chekos AK, Repke JT (2001) Postpartum sexual functioning and its relationship to perineal trauma: a retrospective cohort study of primiparous women. *American Journal of Obstetrics and Gynecology* 184 (5): 881–888; discussion 888–890.

Small R, Lumley J, Donohue L, Potter A, Walderstrom U (2000) Midwife-led debriefing to reduce maternal depression following operative birth: a randomised controlled trial. *British Medical Journal* 321 (7268): 1043–1047.

Smith GCS, Pell JP, Dobbie R (2003) Caesarean section and risk of unexplained stillbirth in subsequent pregnancy. *Lancet* 362: 1779–1784.

Snooks SJ, Setchell M, Swash M, Henry MM (1984) Injury to innervation of pelvic floor sphincter musculature in childbirth. *Lancet* 2 (8402): 546–550.

Sultan AH (1997) Anal incontinence after childbirth. *Current Opinion Obstetrics and Gynecology* 9 (5): 320–324.

Thompson JF, Roberts CL, Currie M, Ellwood DA (2000) Maternal health problems after childbirth: a prospective study. *4th Annual Conference of the Perinatal Society of Australia and New Zealand (PSANZ)*. Brisbane: Perinatal Society of Australia & New Zealand, 49.

Thompson JF, Roberts CL, Currie M, Ellwood DA (2002) Prevalence and persistence of health problems after childbirth: associations with parity and method of birth. *Birth* 29 (2): 83–94.

Van Kessel K, Reed S, Newton K, Meier A, Lentz G (2001) The second stage of labor and stress urinary incontinence. *American Journal of Obstetrics and Gynecology* 184 (7): 1571–1575.

Vendittelli F, Boniol M, Mamelle N (2005) Early postpartum hospital discharge in France. *Revue D'epidemiologie et de Sante Publique* 53 (4): 373–382.

Villar J, Carroli G, Zavaleta N, *et al.* World Health Organization; Global Survey on Maternal and Perinatal Health Research Group (2007) Maternal and neonatal individual risks and benefits associated with caesarean delivery: multicentre prospective study. *British Medical Journal* 335 (7628): 1025.

Villar J, Valladares E, Wojdyla D, *et al.* WHO 2005 Global Survey on Maternal and Perinatal Health Research Group (2006) Caesarean delivery rates and pregnancy outcomes: the 2005 WHO global survey on maternal and perinatal health in Latin America. *Lancet* 367: 1819–1829.

Weaver J (2007) Are there "Unnecessary" cesarean sections? Perceptions of women and obstetricians about cesarean sections of nonclinical indications. *Birth* 34 (1): 32–41.

Weaver J, Statham H, Richards M (2001) High caesarean section rates among women over 30. High rates may be due to perceived potential for complications. *British Medical Journal* 323 (7307): 284–285.

Williams A, Herron-Marx S, Knibb R (2007) The prevalence of enduring post-natal perineal morbidity and its relationship to type of birth and birth risk factors. *Journal of Clinical Nursing* 16: 549–561.

World Health Organization (1998) *Postpartum Care of the Mother and Newborn.* Geneva: A Practical Guide, World Health Organization.

Chapter 7
Baby-Friendly Hospitals: What Can They Achieve?

Val Finigan

Introduction

There are no apologies made for commencing this chapter with this statement: *'Mother's milk will always matter, it will always be the best'* (Minchin 1998).

Benefits of breastfeeding for mother and baby

Current policy in the United Kingdom is to promote exclusive breast-feeding (feeding only breast milk) for the first 6 months of life. It is recommended that breastfeeding should continue for as long as the mother and baby wish, whilst gradually introducing a more varied diet (DoH 2003). Breast milk is a unique and complex collection of nutrients that are necessary for optimal infant development and growth. These nutrients affect the infant metabolically, immunologically and neuro-logically. Babies that are breastfed are provided with complete nutrition and are less likely to become ill in both the short and the long term (Horta *et al.* 2007).

A breastfed baby, in comparison to its formula-fed counterpart, is five times less likely to be hospitalised with gastrointestinal infection regardless of socio-economic conditions, five times less likely to have a urine infection, twice less likely to have a chest or ear infection and if it is from an allergic family it is twice less likely to present with asthma, eczema or insulin-dependent diabetes (Howie *et al.* 1990; Marild *et al.* 1990; Wilson *et al.* 1998; Fewtrell 2004). It is recognised that breastfed infants will become healthier adults with less risks of obesity, coronary heart disease or raised blood pressure (Horta *et al.* 2007).

Mothers who do not breastfeed have double the risks of death from breast cancer under the age of 55 (Short 1994), whilst breastfeeding mothers are protected against ovarian cancer and fractured bones later in their lives (Gwinn *et al.* 1990; Rossenblatt & Thomas 1993; UK National Case Control Study Group 1993; Newcombe *et al.* 1994).

Breastfeeding is not solely about nutrition – it is also about nurture. The close contact between a mother and baby engenders confident parenting and supports the development of an intimate and affection-ate bond between mother and child. Such closeness may be especially important for those living in circumstances of social deprivation and where there is low esteem (NICE 2005). The close skin-to-skin contact and tactile touch displayed during breastfeeding has been shown to enhance development of the emotional part of the infant's brain, reduc-ing later risks of emotional and developmental disorders in infants, for example, attention-deficit disorder (Gerhardt 2006). NICE (2005) recog-nised that there is also a public health question that needs to be asked about the costs related to infant feeding from increased use of resources for families and also for the health service, absence from work related to childhood illness, health risks associated with formula milk feeding both in the short and long term (Minchin 1998) – all have an economic impact on the wider society.

Although many women know about the health benefits of breastfeed-ing (Bolling *et al.* 2007) increasing initiation and duration rates appear difficult. Whilst midwives chant today's prevailing mantra 'Breast is Best', women in maternity units across the United Kingdom continue to report that they feel unsupported when they come to feed their babies (particularly if they are first-time mothers) (Dykes 2006). The culture of health promotion and education in which health professionals operate can profoundly affect the mother's decision in regard to feeding her infant. Perhaps as Hoddinott and Pill (1999) suggest, initially the major-ity of women intend to breastfeed but their early experiences of care are often difficult and off-putting and lead to the demise of that intent. Increased hospitalisation of women during childbirth and the greater demands placed upon overworked and under-resourced midwives are blamed for the poor breastfeeding rates. Thus, the challenge in the United Kingdom is to create a culture in which breastfeeding is seen as the conventional way to feed a baby and to provide the right kind of support within constrained National Health Service (NHS) resources to support women successfully.

In this chapter, the evidence of what helps and hinders the drive to increase breastfeeding rates will be explored. By highlighting an experi-ence of one maternity unit's implementation of the United Nations Chil-dren's Fund (UNICEF) Baby-Friendly programme (UNICEF 1991), the chapter will demonstrate the potential for the emergence of a new maternity culture that is breastfeeding, mother, father and midwife friendly.

Baby feeding in the United Kingdom: what is the current situation?

Despite well-documented evidence on the short- and long-term effects of breastfeeding on infant and maternal well-being, the United Kingdom has one of the highest rates of artificial feeding of newborn babies in the world. In 2000, only 69% of mothers initiated breastfeeding, falling to 52% at 2 weeks, 42% at 6 weeks and 21% at 6 months (Hamlyn *et al.* 2002). The rates have barely shown improvement since 1995 (Table 7.1), although there have been some slight increases among lower-income groups. In 2005, the UK infant feeding survey (Bolling *et al.* 2007) showed that 78% of women in England breastfed their babies, the prevalence of breastfeeding had also increased, but when related to the increased initiation, the proportion of mothers still breastfeeding at 6 weeks (50%) and 6 months (26%) remained the same as in 2000 (UNICEF UK BFI 2005). The median rate of breastfeeding in the United Kingdom is around 1 month, as compared with 5 months or more in other European countries, including Belgium, Switzerland and Denmark (Nicoll *et al.* 2002). Furthermore, 9 out of 10 women who stopped breastfeeding reported that they would have liked to continue for longer, and the reasons for them stopping were on the whole because of poor practices and a lack of support (Bolling 2007).

Acheson's (1998) independent inquiry informed us of the impact of poverty on the health and nutritional status of women and children. The inquiry identified that mothers from disadvantaged groups are more likely than others to give birth to low birth weight babies. Furthermore, the inquiry pointed out that breastfeeding is a strong indicator of social inequalities (disadvantaged population groups are the least likely to breastfeed).

Table 7.1 Breastfeeding rates.

	1980 (%)	1985 (%)	1990 (%)	1995 (%)	2000 (%)	2006 (%)
Birth	65	64	63	68	71	78
1 week	57	55	53	53	55	63
2 weeks	52	51	50		52	
6 weeks	41	38	39	42	42	48
4 months	26	26	25		28	
6 months	22	21	21	21	21	25

Reproduced by kind permission of UNICEF.

There are wide variations between postcode areas reflecting geographical patterns of economic advantage and deprivation (North West Framework for Action 2008). The infant feeding survey (Bolling 2007) confirmed that low maternal age, low educational attainment and low socio-economic position continue to impact on infant feeding patterns. For example, 65% of UK women in managerial and professional occupations were breastfeeding at 6 weeks compared to only 32% of those from routine and manual groups. The government (DoH 1999) recognised that infant feeding practices were an issue related to inequity and this public health issue was underlined in the government's NHS Plan (DoH 2000) where a reduction of health inequalities was requested. It was noted that lower levels of breastfeeding contributed to increased morbidities in lower socio-economic groups, with particular reference to cancers, obesity and coronary heart disease.

Mothers living on low incomes have diverse reasons for not initiating and sustaining breastfeeding and the Department of Health has charged local health authorities with increasing the rates in these groups by 2% points year upon year (DoH 2002). Real and sustainable rises in the breastfeeding rates within these groups will have the greatest benefits reducing morbidity and mortality in infants and narrowing the inequalities gap in both nutrition and health (DoH 2003).

Improving breastfeeding rates: what works?

Whilst surveys have tended to show that the mother's age, level of education and social class are strongly associated with the choice of feeding method (Hamlyn *et al.* 2002; Bolling *et al.* 2007), other studies have been carried out using qualitative methods and have looked deeper, uncovering indicators that the surveys could not (Hoddinott & Pill 1999; Earle 2002; Mahon-Daly & Andrews 2002). These studies have shown the impact of everyday cultures on women's experiences and expectations of feeding their infants. The cultural aspects of breastfeeding are underpinned by beliefs, attitudes, practices and social structures of everyday life. Feeding decisions are never made in isolation; they are discovered and influenced by notions of sexuality, embarrassment of feeding in public, the healthcare system, and cultural messages that formula feeding is the norm and that breastfeeding is not what normal women do (Bailey *et al.* 2004). The social 'norm' has been shown to be a strong determinant in the decisions of individuals to perform or not to perform health behaviours (Fishbein & Ajzen 1975). Women on the whole continue to lack confidence in their ability to breastfeed and in particular, their capacity to provide sufficient milk for their babies (Dykes & Williams 1999; Dykes 2002). A study examining the attitudes of school children aged 11 found that they saw breastfeeding to be embarrassing and bottle-feeding to be convenient and fashionable (Gregg 1989). Furthermore the social and physical support given to breastfeeding women by family members including their partners has been associated with increased levels of breastfeeding initiation and continuation (Scott & Binns 1999). Disrupting the strong cycles of beliefs will be difficult and will need a multifaceted and targeted approach (NICE 2008). This approach will include health education interventions, health sector initiatives, peer support programmes and media campaigns – all aimed to affect the way families are socialised in order to shift the culture.

NICE (2005) carried out a systematic review of public health interventions to promote the duration of breastfeeding and the main finding highlighted the huge gap in knowledge that existed in relation to what worked in disadvantaged population groups. NICE (2005) also showed a gap in the evidence base relating to ascertaining the views of child-bearing women and their families, and the staff who cared for them, whose voices were largely silent in relation to interventions that may be effective. NICE (2005) was, however, able to show interventions that were effective or ineffective at that time. These included skilled breastfeeding support, peer or professional support proactively being offered to women who wanted to breastfeed (Dennis 2002; Porteous *et al.* 2000) and the implementation of the UNICEF Baby-Friendly Hospital Initiative (BFHI) in both acute and primary healthcare settings. A barrier to implementation of this programme is the costs, but the costs are minimal in comparison to the costs of treating the ill health linked to not breastfeeding.

Peer support

NICE (2005) found high-quality evidence that both health professional and peer support can be effective in supporting both exclusive and any breastfeeding, suggesting that a coordinated approach between hospitals and local communities is needed. Numerous descriptive studies suggest that peer support is an effective strategy for increasing breast-feeding rates (Kisten *et al.* 1994; Gross *et al.* 1998; Penrose *et al.* 1998; NICE 2005, 2008). The impact of peer support on breastfeeding depends upon the background and training of the counsellor and the interaction between the counsellor and her clients (CAPC/CPNP 2001). Sikorski and Renfrew's (1999) analysis of studies reported that predominantly, face-to-face support has a benefit whilst peer programmes that rely on telephone contacts alone do not.

Peer support is especially necessary in countries that have a strong bottle-feeding culture like the United Kingdom. There appears to have been a loss of community-based, woman-centred, embodied and experiential knowledge related to breastfeeding (Dykes 2006). This loss has created a need to develop mother-to-mother support. Yet, many types of breastfeeding support are already currently available, for example, support from a wide range of healthcare professionals, public health nurses, lactation consultants and voluntary supporters trained by organisations with established accreditation programmes (Association of Breastfeeding mothers, La Leche League, National Childbirth Trust and the Breastfeeding Network). What remains challenging for the NHS is to find out what programmes are most effective in different areas of the United Kingdom, what the cost of providing different support for breastfeeding women is, whether the NHS can afford peer programmes and if, and when, peer support should be made available in each different community setting.

There are differences amongst the diverse voluntary training programmes but the fundamental approach is woman centred and nondirective; it is about empowering the woman to make her own decision, providing her with information and knowledge to inform that decision and being skilled enough to listen and counsel her. According to Dykes (2006) the training for lay supporters has a strong reflexive component allowing trainees to debrief their own experiences along the way. Trainees learn person-centred counselling skills, empathetic understanding, unconditional positive regard (non-judgmental acceptance) and genuineness (Rogers 1961).

Although Sirkoski and Renfrew (1999) argue that there may be no difference between paid or volunteer peer support, this certainly has not been evaluated. Atkins (2008), the founder of 'Little Angels' in Blackburn (see Chapter 5), feels that payment for peer breastfeeding supporters is of paramount importance and highlights that breastfeeding support is skilled work and is of value to the society and that payment acknowledges its value. Furthermore, Atkins (2008) suggests that peer support is something that needs to be managed and evaluated if it is going to be successful. Anecdotal feedback (North West Breastfeeding Liaison Group 2008) supports this view, seeing the maintenance of unpaid and unmanaged peer support to be challenging and often ineffective. Whilst women on the whole are altruistic and willingly seek to help others by becoming breastfeeding supporters, the compelling need to return to work early leaves them unable to commit the time to use their new-found skill effectively. The financial and resource effects on services of providing in-depth and time-consuming training and then in essence 'getting nothing in return' leaves women offering these services disgruntled. However, it could be argued that the skill is never lost or wasted, and women trained to become peer supporters often use their skill to influence breastfeeding in their workplaces or in their home environment with their friends and neighbours. Furthermore, gaining a qualification provides the stepping stone to employment, and this is debated further in Chapter 5.

Professional support

One of the many and complex factors contributing to low breastfeeding rates in the United Kingdom is the lack of education and preparation of health practitioners to effectively support breastfeeding (Renfrew *et al.* 2005). This is in spite of the compelling evidence that their knowledge and skill can be paramount in promoting breastfeeding (Renfrew *et al.* 2005). Evidence from the United Kingdom indicates that women experience inconsistent information and inappropriate attitudes from healthcare professionals (Simmons 2003; McFadden *et al.* 2006; Smale *et al.* 2006). It could be suggested that this lack of skills and knowledge may place women at risk of harm. Recommendations for training and updating healthcare professionals about breastfeeding have been put forward (Audit Commission 1997). Encouragingly, there is evidence that good practice breastfeeding education can be effective in improving the care women are offered. The main training courses currently available in the United Kingdom include those offered by the BFHI, and evidence suggests that these programmes are effective (Valdes *et al.* 1995; Hall Moran *et al.* 2000). Furthermore, improving breastfeeding knowledge and skills of practitioners has the potential to have a substantial impact on breastfeeding communities that have a low prevalence of breastfeeding (Dykes 2003), and women in these communities have the most health benefits to gain from breastfeeding.

The Baby-friendly initiative in the United Kingdom – good for baby, mother and midwife

Since the 1970s, the Department of Health has acknowledged the need to halt the decline in breastfeeding initiation and duration by improving support offered to women during their maternity care (DHSS 1974). In 1993, the UNICEF BFHI was launched and introduced within the United Kingdom for this purpose (Woolridge 1994). The initiative is based on the Ten Steps to successful breastfeeding, research-based practices that intend to promote, protect and support breastfeeding and also the implementation of the International Code of Marketing of Breastmilk Substitutes (WHO 1981; UNICEF 2008). The programme is backed by an external assessment and award programme (Table 7.2).

Similar values have been developed for community services in the '7-point plan' (UNICEF UK BFI 1998) and for paediatric units (Shore *et al.* 1998). In addition, there are standards for educational facilities providing appropriate training for healthcare staff (UNICEF 2007). These standards aim to ensure that health professionals are trained in breastfeeding, have the right skills and knowledge to support women and are able to implement changes directed within policies, from the

Table 7.2 Geographical breastfeeding rates.

Hospital name	Pre-BFI rates (%)	BFI rates (%)
Royal Oldham Hospital	29 (1994)	66 (2007)
North Manchester general	29 (1999)	62 (2007)
Blackburn	27 (1997)	72 (2007)
Bradford	53 (1999)	62 (2004)
Glasgow	51 (1997)	67 (2004)
Derby	50 (1996)	72 (2004)
Halifax	65 (1995)	74 (2004)

start of their careers. Evidence suggests that skilled health professionals positively influence breastfeeding women (Humenick *et al.* 1998), yet in the United Kingdom conflicting information and advice remains common within healthcare settings, causing confusion and undermining women's confidence (Garcia *et al.* 1998; Tarkka *et al.* 1998; Dykes & Williams 1999; Dykes 2005).

The drive to implement and achieve UNICEF 'Baby-Friendly' status has never been more compelling. In England, it has been recommended that purchasers should incorporate the Ten Steps into their commissioning plans (DOH 1995; NICE 2006a), thereby embedding the evidence base into the mainstream of health and social services in the United Kingdom. However, many service providers continue to ignore this recommendation as the pull on finite budgets is challenging, and expenditure linked to health promotion is given low priority. Although heath and social care targets are highlighting breastfeeding as a key achievement (DoH 2002) and monitoring is in place to ensure an upward trend in rates, there continues to be a reluctance in some areas to implement the BFHI standards.

The culture of maternity services can and does profoundly influence new mothers' decisions of how to feed their infants. If services are not supportive of breastfeeding even the most committed mother may not succeed. Research on infant feeding policies in maternity wards (Perez-Escamilla *et al.* 1994) identified factors in maternity units that impact breastfeeding success. This research underpins the UNICEF Baby-Friendly initiative and the full research is summarised in a related document (WHO 1998).

Wright (1998) suggests that the implementation of the BFHI involves deliberately unsettling the medicalised culture that has evolved in maternity care over the last century, but Dykes (2006) is concerned that in doing so we may merely be exchanging one dominant culture (medicalisation) for another, without addressing the constraints that are placed upon women to maintain breastfeeding in today's society. Women on the whole are part of the paid workforce and workplace policies to support exclusive breastfeeding for up to 6 months, and breastfeeding beyond this point rarely exists. To compound women's issues further, the predominant bottle-feeding culture within the United Kingdom, the strong marketing of breast milk substitutes and the difficulty of breastfeeding in public may all present a dissonance for women. Breastfeeding continues to be portrayed in the media and experienced by many women, particularly those from socially deprived communities, as a marginal and liminal activity, rarely seen and barely spoken about (Hoddinott & Pill 1999). Thus, for many women breastfeeding takes place in secret, hidden from others in order to cover up their embarrassment and sexuality. Vogel and Mitchell (1998) suggest that in an attempt to protect women, they should be supported to learn to breastfeed comfortably in front of others (if culturally acceptable) prior to having to do so in the real situation. Healthcare professionals and peer supporters can positively influence a woman's confidence and skills in breastfeeding, by simply spending time and making themselves available to teach them and support them to breastfeed successfully using an approach that requires no or minimal contact (hands-off approach). The challenge for healthcare professionals is to facilitate women to explore their own knowledge and problem-solving abilities rather than merely doing what we have always done and telling mothers what to do or doing it for them (Whelan & Lupton 1998). This participative model of care is described further in Chapter 5.

The NICE (2008) health guidance also recognised that a multifaceted approach or a coordinated programme across different settings maximises the potential for increased breastfeeding rates. The strategies include raising awareness of the health benefits of breastfeeding for both mother and baby during pregnancy, policy production based on current available evidence, training for healthcare staff, peer-support breastfeeding programmes and support with breastfeeding in the postnatal period for mothers as influencing factors. There is strong evidence that demonstrates that adopting BFHI improves breastfeeding initiation rates and increases hospital staff awareness, knowledge and skills empowering them (Kramer *et al.* 2001; Philipp *et al.* 2003; Broadfoot *et al.* 2005), and new national guidance on postnatal care (NICE 2006b) directs NHS organisations to adopt a programme of education and support such as BFHI in its six key core recommendations (described in the subsequent text).

The Baby-Friendly accreditation process is undertaken in stages (Box 7.1). Trusts that are successful are then re-assessed at frequent intervals to ensure that compliance with the UNICEF principles are maintained and embedded into the culture of services.

Box 7.1 UNICEF Baby-Friendly stages

Register intent
Action planning visit
Certificate of commitment awarded
Stage 1 – submit paper work for review
Stage 2 – staff knowledge and skills audited by UNICEF
Stage 3 – assessment by UNICEF for full accreditation (involves paper-
    work, staff, clients and endorsement of WHO code 'marketing of breast
    milk substitutes')
Reproduced by kind permission of UNICEF.

Many healthcare professionals remain concerned that implementation of the UNICEF standards will take away women's choice and cause them to feel guilty if they chose to bottle-feed. It is important then to reinforce the fact that the BFHI is clearly focused upon supporting informed choice and aims to provide an equitable service once a decision has been made. The BFHI does not intend to be coercive or to place any pressure on women to breastfeed; rather, it has been developed to be protective of mothers who have chosen to breastfeed.

The BFHI has played the role of challenger by opening up health systems to the scrutiny and judgment of their users. Murray (1994) suggests that the BFHI is a recipe for empowerment, providing access to facts and information, the right to informed choice and real options from which to choose.

Although the Ten Steps (Box 7.2) appear simple on first consideration, implementation in the United Kingdom has been fraught with difficulties, as instigating the standards requires a shift in both health professionals' culture and in their routines. Thus, for people leading such a fundamental change in practice, it becomes clear that they must be able to empower both professionals and mothers alike. Equipping clinicians with appropriate skills and knowledge, applying the evidence in a multifaceted and integrated manner, overcoming a likely climate of limited resources and being truly passionate about the promotion of breastfeeding can lead to success (Dykes 1995, 2005; HDA 2003; Calvert 2005).

Box 7.2 UNICEF Ten Steps

1. Have a written breastfeeding policy that is routinely communicated to all
   healthcare staff.
2. Train all healthcare staff in skills necessary to implement this policy.
3. Inform all pregnant women about the benefits and management of breastfeeding.

4. Help mothers initiate breastfeeding within half-hour of birth.
5. Show mothers how to breastfeed and how to maintain lactation, even if they are separated from their infants.
6. Give newborn infants no food or drink other than breast milk, unless medically indicated.
7. Practice rooming-in – allow mothers and infants to remain together – 24 hours a day.
8. Encourage breastfeeding on demand.
9. Give no artificial teats or pacifiers (also called dummies) to breastfeeding infants.
10. Foster the establishment of breastfeeding support groups and refer mothers to them on discharge from the hospital or clinic.
Reproduced by kind permission of UNICEF.

It is important to consider the notable effects on breastfeeding initiation from the implementation of the UNICEF standards. In units that have achieved success there are remarkable improvements in the breastfeeding rates (NICE 2006c). It has been estimated that units engaging in the UNICEF programme will increase the initiation of breastfeeding by a minimum of 10.6% over a 4-year period (NICE 2006c) and that this improvement is sustainable. The hospitals that were reported within the NICE 'Postnatal Guidance' (2006b) all had high deprivation scores and higher-than-average levels of ethnicity and teenage pregnancies (NICE 2006c) – factors that have increased the challenges associated with implementing UNICEF's standards.

Why is it good for the mother, the baby and the midwife?

Care provided in the baby-friendly way can engender more baby-friendly mother care; the mother's confidence in her ability to nurture is developed right from the moment of birth. In this critical period, the baby is placed close to its mother and the midwife empowers her to care for and get to know her newborn baby. Researchers and psychoanalysts have recognised that reciprocal behaviour between a mother and her baby is crucial for breastfeeding, for attachment and also for the baby's brain development (Dechateau & Wiberg 1977; Wiberg *et al.* 1989; Righard & Alade 1990; Christensson *et al.* 1995; Finigan & Davies 2004; Gerhardt 2006).

Gerhardt (2006) proposes that babies are born with adequate brain neurons to last their entire lives. However, she purports that the synapses between neurons develop during the first 2 years of life, in response to touch and massage. Scan pictures show that when reciprocal behaviour is carried out, synapses become dense and, in particular, denser in those areas that govern emotional being. Where babies are not touched as much, the developments of synapses within the emotional regions of the brain are sparse. Gerhardt puts forward that the growing problems seen in today's society with children displaying behavioural problems may be generated simply from a lack of loving touch and reciprocal responsiveness early in life.

It has been suggested that 'Baby-Friendly Hospital' also equates to Baby-Friendly mothers (Murray 1994; Gerhardt 2006). For example, adoption of step 4 means mothers are encouraged to use skin contact with their babies for nurturing and also to encourage breastfeeding, and it has been recognised that skin-to-skin contact has a positive effect on the babies' growth, health and emotional development throughout life (Montagu 1986; Murray 1994; Odent 2003; Finigan & Davies 2004; Kroeger & Smith 2004; Gerhardt 2006). Implementation of the standards appears to also engender more confident mothering and successful and natural breastfeeding (Odent 2003; Finigan & Davies 2004).

Dykes (2000) suggests that when healthcare professionals have a sound working knowledge of the principles of basic person-centred counselling and a concomitant knowledge of the principles underpinning effective breastfeeding, they will be empowered and feel enthusiastic and committed to assist women. Furthermore, with the right skills and knowledge they will be able to use evidence-based practices appropriately.

Dykes (2006) posits that investing in a specialist (who crosses the hospital–community interface) to act as a resource for staff and a support for service users will aid services to effectively implement the changes required for UNICEF Baby-Friendly accreditation. This coordinator needs senior status and management of change capabilities (Broome 1998).

Experience of implementing the UNICEF standards: a success story

Being involved in the change management required to achieve 'Baby-Friendly' practices highlights the fact that it is not an easy task and is somewhat challenging. However, once the standard is achieved there is a tremendous pride within the organisation and this contributes to a positive corporate culture. The Pennine Acute NHS Hospitals Trust, Blackburn, Derby, Bradford and Halifax hospitals are all good examples of the success of the BFHI. All of these hospitals serve populations with higher-than-average deprivation scores, and the deprivation in the northeast sector of Greater Manchester is clearly linked to the increased minority ethnic populations, pockets of social deprivation and higher-than-average levels of adolescent pregnancy. In the northeast sector of Greater Manchester, the breastfeeding initiation rate is below the national standards (Table 7.2). However, the area's organisational strategic aims show a commitment to improve the health of the local population and to reduce health inequalities by altering the culture.

One hospital in the northwest of England implemented the UNICEF BFHI standards and showed improved breastfeeding rates. In 1994, 29% of women began to breastfeed their babies but before they were discharged from the maternity unit almost all of them had stopped. The reasons given were sore nipples, frequent feeding, unsettled babies and too little or poor-quality milk. It was noted that all of the above could be addressed by an improvement in professional practice.

The journey began by identifying a leader who had a passion to support women to breastfeed successfully. Future prospects for the leader would involve managing a fundamental change in practice. This task was daunting, but 'anybody can change things, you make a difference if you feel it's worthwhile and if you really care, it's the belief that's important' (Palmer 2003). Whilst the challenge of becoming Baby Friendly can seem overwhelming, a belief in the philosophy underpinning the programme can enhance the potential for success.

Champions (i.e. staff members who were interested and passionate about breastfeeding) were crucial to the success of the programme. The team of champions was made familiar with the BFHI and each staff member was relied upon to influence and assist in directing the changes required within their individual working areas, giving them ownership of the change.

Step 1: A written breastfeeding policy

The programme expects a breastfeeding policy for staff and parents. A multidisciplinary team formulated the breastfeeding policy and a consultative process followed in order for all medical, midwifery and nursing staff to agree to its contents and have ownership. A joint policy was designed for both acute and primary care settings. The policy was based on current evidence and was freely available for both mothers and staff, either as a written document or via the Trust's intranet system.

Step 2: Staff education

The Ten Steps were used to formulate a staff-training programme for all levels of staff, from the ward cleaners to consultant staff, as anyone who came into contact with breastfeeding women and their babies required some level of guidance. Dykes (2006) states that knowledge comes from a variety of sources: embodied knowledge (subjective, acquired through personal experiences and perceptions of breastfeeding a baby); vicarious knowledge (general learning generated throughout life, seeing others breastfeed); practice-based knowledge (learned by observation of others) and formal theoretical knowledge (structured learning opportunities within education). Each aspect of learning must be addressed within the educational package for professionals if it is to be successful.

The 18-hour training requirement from UNICEF may be a stumbling block for many organisations, yet it is essential if breastfeeding practices are to improve. This challenge could be overcome by having a practical workshop that takes place over a 5-hour period, focused on developing and enhancing skills for breastfeeding and taught in an innovative and user-friendly way. Completing a workbook equates to a further 5 hours and provides the theory that underpins the practical session. Clinical supervision and ward-based reflective sessions meet the remaining 8 hours of the 18-hour programme.

Locally for the author, this training was made mandatory on an annual basis. Supervised practice was crucial, as some staff had never seen a woman or a baby breastfeed and were unaware of the different positions that could be used and why positioning and attachment were so important. The sessions empowered staff to consider all aspects of their care, and helped them to realise that the mother must be the 'expert' and that they needed to support her in an unobtrusive and gentle way.

A separate programme was designed and delivered to medical staff on a bi-annual basis and equates to 1 hour of study. In the past, there had been little or no education provided for medical staff, and to our surprise, most of them welcomed the sessions.

All training is monitored and evaluated on a database, with supervisors of midwives and managers being informed annually of attendance, as it is their responsibility to ensure staff compliance.

Step 3: Antenatal information

Antenatal workshops, breastfeeding sessions in parent-craft and antenatal checklists of information given were developed. The curriculum for antenatal education includes the health benefits of breastfeeding, breastfeeding in hospitals, the benefits of having skin-to-skin contact at birth, rooming-in and baby-led feeding, coping with contradictory advice, support systems for successful and enjoyable breastfeeding and managing early challenges. The checklist and patient interviews enable an audit of this standard and the results are fed back on a frequent basis so that staff can see that they are achieving the standard or what needs to be improved.

Step 4: Skin-to-skin contact

The importance of keeping mothers and babies together is paramount, whether mothers choose to breastfeed or not. Midwives are aware of the evidence supporting the effects of skin-to-skin contact, for example, the thermo-regulation that occurs between mother and baby (Christensson *et al.* 1992) that skin contact stabilises the baby's heart and respiratory rate (Lagercrantz & Slotkin 1986; Christensson *et al.* 1995) and that early breastfeeding takes place. The baby becomes colonised against bacteria from the mother's home environment which are prevalent in her skin flora at the time of birth (Christensson *et al.* 1992). Midwives encourage mothers to keep their babies in close skin contact following birth for even longer periods than those recommended by UNICEF, particularly if the baby has not initiated breastfeeding within the first hour of birth. Midwives recognise that their workload is likely to be more if a baby has not fed early and is separated from its mother.

Step 5: Show women how to breastfeed and maintain their lactation if separated from their babies

This step focuses on staff skills, to support the ability for them to use a hands-off-mother approach to teach new mothers how to breastfeed independently. Staff must also be skilled in hand expression and in teaching the mother this skill, so that she is self-reliant. If the baby has to be separated from its mother, the mother will be advised to hand-express or use a pump at least eight times in 24 hours, with one of those times being at night. Prolactin, the milk-producing hormone, is known to peak from midnight, so expression of milk after this time will increase the milk yield the following day (Riordan 2005). The mother is less likely to wake up with engorged breasts if she has expressed her milk during the night.

Step 6: Give breastfed babies no food or drink other than their mother's breast milk

Staff may have a poor understanding of why this information is important, and implementation can be challenging. Educating staff and women through raising awareness of the effects of supplementary feeds helps enormously. Supplementary feeds affect the immature infant's immune system and increase the risks of infection (Howie *et al.* 1990), which is so important in local populations where there is a high incidence of asthma, eczema and diabetes, and the literature demonstrates that this sensitivity to allergens has been traced to early and complimentary artificial milk feeds (Pettitt *et al.* 1997; Minchin 1998; Paronen *et al.* 2000). Apart from the obvious health risks, the effect on the mother's lactation needs to be given recognition. The mother's confidence in her milk production or even the quality of her milk may be undermined when supplements are offered. A baby that has received formula milk is less likely to be satisfied with the small volume of milk the breasts produce in the early days. If a mother does not feed her baby then her breasts may become overfull. Increase in a protein within the milk (feedback inhibitor of lactation) when breasts are left full for a period of time may diminish the mother's lactation, and this can be either a short- or a long-term effect (Riordan 2005).

Step 7: Rooming-in

Rooming-in ensures confident mothering (Ekström *et al.* 2005) as the mother learns to pick up and respond to her baby's cues. Most staff were happy to see the withdrawal of the use of nurseries and the babies next to their mothers.

The use of clip-on-cots on the postnatal ward has assisted in the success of achieving this standard. The postnatal ward is not suitable for co-sleeping (Ball *et al.* 2006) and studies suggest that babies in clip-on-cots feed as frequently as those that do bed-share and co-sleep with their mothers (Ball *et al.* 2006). The Trust's decision to provide the cots has shown their commitment to the Baby-Friendly status and also to breastfeeding. The mothers articulate that they like the cots as they can self-care and do not have to rely on staff members to pass their babies to them. They can respond to their babies' early cues for feeding and feel better that their babies are not crying and keeping other mothers and babies awake.

Step 8: Demand feeding

Encouraging breastfeeding on demand is an accepted postnatal ward practice. The mothers and staff are made aware of the baby's physiology and expected feeding pattern. The mother quickly becomes the connoisseur, responsive to her baby's early signs for feeding. Healthcare workers and mothers are frequently surprised to find out that the baby's stomach capacity at birth is 9 ml in total and that during day 1 of motherhood the breasts produce approximately 7 ml of colostrum per feed (38 ml per first 24 hours of feeding), (Hartmann *et al.* 1995). It is somewhat perplexing when one considers that artificially fed babies are encouraged to drink as much as 20 or 30 ml of formula milk with a tougher curd at this same time. Such practice helps us to see the link between artificial feeding and obesity, with bottle-fed babies being heavier and larger than their breastfed counterparts at 1 year of age (Riordan 2005; WHO 2007).

Step 9: Give no teats, dummies or pacifiers to breastfed babies

This step establishes that no teats or dummies should be given to breastfed babies. Changing culture is never an easy task and dummies have been used for many years, with, almost 80% of babies given one to pacify them (Howard *et al.* 2003). The use of dummies is more common in populations of lower socio-economic status (Mathur *et al.* 1990). What becomes clear is that if we are to meet the challenge of this step then mothers need to be made aware of other ways that they can settle their babies, for example, rocking, containment holding and skin-to-skin contact.

All interventions should have a solid rationale and research basis before becoming recommended practice by healthcare professionals. Given that there is a lack of evidence of benefit and a wide and diverse documented risk associated with the use of dummies (Howard *et al.* 2003), parents should be cautioned to avoid them during early breastfeeding. The 'social' use of dummies has been linked to dental and orthodontic problems (Drane 1996) and to accidents such as choking, increased risks of thrush and other infections (Mattos-Graner *et al.* 2001). Lehtonen (1998) suggests that dummies can affect speech and developmental progress, and furthermore a baby that is sucking on a dummy will have limited periods of suckling at the breast and this may consequently affect milk drainage and thus limit milk production (Aarts *et al.* 1999).

Mothers who wish to use a dummy or teat in the early period should be informed that use in the first 4 weeks of life may affect breast milk production and potentially could cause breast refusal. During this time, both the mother and her baby are learning the art and skill of breastfeeding and it is important that nothing interferes with their learning. However, if a mother chooses to use a dummy she should be told not to withdraw it suddenly and to put the baby to sleep with a dummy at each occurrence in line with the recent guidance on risks of Sudden Infant Death Syndrome (Hauck *et al.* 2005).

Step 10: Establish support groups and refer mothers to them

Breastfeeding support groups, both volunteer and professional, should be available and mothers should be told about them while in hospital. Women need to know where they can get help in order to continue to breastfeed when they meet challenges and for access to social support.

Evidence/costing

The NICE (2006a) states that there is no cost-effectiveness studies that deal with the BFHI in England and Wales. However, they did take into account evidence provided by eight maternity units regarding their experiences of implementing Baby-Friendly Initiative (BFI) initiation rates prior and after implementation, and relevant demographics were collected. In addition, NICE used information from one unit in Northern Ireland and data from one hospital in Glasgow. This evidence was used to direct the NICE guidance that the BFI should be a minimum core recommendation for maternity services because it is likely that it is cost-effective (NICE 2006a).

At the time of the NICE analysis, England and Wales had 34 accredited units, 58 units with a certificate of commitment and 183 un-accredited units. Today across the United Kingdom, there are 21 (4 with accreditation suspended) BFHI maternity units and 57 maternity units holding a certificate of commitment (UNICEF 2007). However, BFHI uptake appears to be a 'postcode lottery' in that a baby born in Scotland will have almost a 59% chance of being in a BFHI accredited unit; in the North of England there is approximately a 25% chance, whilst in the South of England it is unlikely that the unit will be BFHI accredited at all (UNICEF 2007).

It is difficult to judge the financial costs of implementation, as different units will implement the standards in very different ways, for example, the costs of training staff was analysed within the NICE guidance and was estimated by using the training programme from one unit in east Lancashire. This unit provides a whole 2-day course for new starters. In comparison, other units provide training in different ways, for example, using short workshops with accompanying workbooks and clinical supervised practices on the wards, and this may be more cost-effective. NICE estimated the cost of implementing BFHI at £7.825 million over a 15-year period (NICE 2006b) 208.

In contrast, NICE also evaluated the cost-effectiveness associated with the implementation of the BFHI. Breastfeeding rates are significantly altered as trusts implement the standards and this in itself may reduce costs on other parts of the health service. Information from UNICEF identified that those units that do implement the standards see an average increase in their breastfeeding rates of 11% over a 4-year period compared to the national trend seen in the triennial reports. Cost assumptions on an increase in breastfeeding of 11% are estimated to save approximately £5 million per annum (for just three illnesses: otitis media, asthma and gastroenteritis). The reduction in maternal and childhood illnesses that are associated with formula milk feeding outweighs the costs of implementation.

This still does not take into account the costs of savings from not purchasing formula milks and teats, costs of other diseases, for example, coronary heart disease, diabetes, eczema, Crohn's disease, or the costs of illness in the mother, for example, ovarian cancer, breast cancer and osteoporosis.

Tappin (1997) suggests that the potential savings for a minimum gain of 2% breastfeeding increase at 6 weeks based on 10 000 births in Glasgow for pre-menopausal breast cancer would save £1000 whilst a 10% increase at 6 weeks would save £4000. Costs associated with diabetes mellitus identify that a 2% increase at 6 weeks which would save £19 000 whilst a 10% increase at the same time would save £98 000. Tappin (1997) also predicted the cost incurred for the potentially life-threatening condition for vulnerable premature infants neonatal necrotising enterocolitis (NEC). Tappin (1997) calculated the savings per 10 cases, finding that giving breast milk to 60% of premature babies would avert four cases of NEC, saving £20 000, and if 100% of premature babies received nothing but breast milk, eight cases would be prevented with a saving of £40 000. In England, a hundred premature lives per year are lost from this condition alone; perhaps it is time to consider offering mother's milk or donated breast milk to all vulnerable babies. Furthermore, the emotional costs to a family can never be measured.

Other public health questions remain about the wider costs related to infant feeding, for example, women who feed their babies formula milk will have more absence from work related to childhood illnesses than their breastfeeding counterparts, and the negative impact of long-term population health will be greater in populations of formula milk-fed infants.

Conclusion

The prevailing strong bottle-feeding culture undermines the initiation of breastfeeding in a number of ways – the feeling of difference engendered by being a breastfeeding mother; the lack of expertise and support amongst both formal and informal networks; the lack of confidence in breastfeeding and the well-established 'rules' that bottle-feeding is the 'norm' and the easiest way to feed a baby. Yet, mothers report that they want consistent advice and skilled support to enable them to breastfeed successfully and for longer periods of time (Hamlyn *et al.* 2002). It can be suggested that mothers generally want to do the best for their babies and that they are beginning to understand the immense health benefits of breastfeeding. Many do their best to give this healthy start in life to their babies, yet this commitment is often undermined by professional practice.

Supporting continued breastfeeding through implementing a multifaceted approach that aims to facilitate both appropriate structural change within the healthcare system and micro-level change within the individual (Dykes 2006) may be most effective. The interventions needed for this approach are those demonstrated within the UNICEF Baby-Friendly hospital and community programmes, training for multidisciplinary staff, subsequent policy and practice changes, culturally appropriate education and peer support programmes, community media activities based on community empowerment (Robertson & Minkler 1994) and social marketing techniques.

If midwives are to contribute to promoting, protecting and supporting breastfeeding, the adoption of the UNICEF Baby-Friendly initiative provides a framework to assist them. Although implementing UNICEF standards is a challenging process, organisations that have achieved this prestigious award feel a sense of pride, which resonates through enhanced staff morale. This enhances the opportunity for women to breastfeed for longer periods of time and staff feeling that they are equipped with the right skills and knowledge to help them. Implementing Baby-Friendly standards demonstrates the commitment of organisations to improving the health of local population groups and to reduce health inequalities.

Key implications for midwifery practice

- Implementing UNICEF Baby-Friendly standards leads to increased breastfeeding rates and is likely to be cost-effective.
- The UNICEF programme empowers midwives, healthcare professionals and mothers.
- Managed, paid, peer breastfeeding support is effective in increasing and sustaining breastfeeding.
- Do you know the inequality gaps in your area of practice? Consider ways in which you may help to narrow those gaps.
- Reflect on the ways in which current hospital practices may impact upon breastfeeding initiation rates and impact upon women's choices.
- Consider how different cultures and society affect women's feeding choices and think of ways that the culture can be altered to accommodate exclusive breastfeeding.

References

Aarts C, Kylberg E, Hornell A, Hofvander Y, Gebre-Medhin M, Greiner T (1999) Breastfeeding patterns in relation to thumb sucking and pacifier use. *Paediatrics* 104: e50.

Acheson D (1998) *Independent Inquiry into Inequalities in Health Reform.* London: The Stationary Office.

Atkins M (2008) Green and Gold the Value of Breastfeeding. Little Angels Conference. Conference Hall Blackburn.

Audit Commission (1997) *First Class Delivery: Improving Maternity Services in England and Wales.* London: Audit Commission.

Ball H, Ward-Platt M, Heslop E, Leech S, Brown K (2006) Infant sleep location the postnatal ward. *Archives of Disease in Childhood.* doi: 10.1136/adc.2006.099416.

Bailey C, Pain RH, Aarvold JE (2004) A give a go breastfeeding culture and early cessation among low income mothers. *Midwifery* 20 (3): 240–250, Elsevier.

Bolling K, Grant C, Hamlyn B, Thornton A (2007) *Infant Feeding Survey.* London: NHS.

Broadfoot M, Britten J, Tappin DM (2005) The baby friendly hospital initiative and breastfeeding rates in Scotland. *Archives of Disease in Childhood Fetal and Neonatal Edition* 90: 114–116.

Broome A (1998) *Managing Change.* London: Macmillan Press LTD.

Calvert J (2005) Strategic planning: the Northern Ireland experience: changing health care practice to improve breastfeeding rates. *UNICEF Annual Conference Notes.* Bournemouth International Centre. November 2005.

CAPC/CPNP (2001) *Think Tank: Factors that Contribute to Increased Breastfeeding in the CAPC/CPNP Population.*

Christensson K, Cabera T, Christensson E, Uvnas-Moberg K, Winberg J (1995) Separation distress call in the neonate in the absence of maternal body contact. *Acta Paediatrica* 84: 468–473.

Christensson K, Siles C, Morenol L (1992) Temperature, metabolic adaptation and crying in healthy full term newborns cared for in skin-to-skin or in a cot. *Acta Paediatrica* 81: 448–493.

Dechateau P, Wiberg B (1977) Long-term effect on mother-infant behaviour of extra contact during the first hour post-partum. *Acta-Paediatrica Scandinavica* 66: 13–151.

Dennis CL (2002) Breastfeeding initiation and duration: a 1990–2000 literature review. *Journal Obstetrics and Gynaecology Neonatal Nursing* 31: 12–32.

Department of Health; National Breastfeeding Working Group (1995) *Breastfeeding: Good Practice Guidance to the NHS.* London: DOH.

Department of Health (1999) *Saving Lives: Our Healthier Nation.* London: Stationary Office.

Department of Health (2000) *The NHS Plan: A Plan for Investment a Plan for Reform.* London: DoH.

Department of Health (2002) *Improvement, Expansion and Reform-the Next Three Years. Priorities and Planning Framework. 2003–2006.* London: DOH.

Department of Health (2003) *Infant Feeding Recommendations.* Available at www.dh.gov:uk/en/publicationsandstatistics/Publications/ PublicationsPolicyAndGuidance/DH4097197 (online accessed 12/07/09).

Department of Health and Social Security (DHSS) (1974) *Present Day Practice in Infant Feeding.* Report of a Working Party of the Panel on Child Nutrition Committee on Medical Aspects of Food Policy. London: HMSO.

Drane D (1996) The effect of teats and dummies on oro-facial development. Presented at: *National Conference of the Australian Lactation Consultants Association*. Hobart, Australia.

Dykes F (1995) Valuing breastfeeding in midwifery education. *British Journal of Midwifery* 3 (10): 544–547.

Dykes F (2002) Western marketing and medicine-construction of an insufficient milk syndrome. *Health Care for Women International* 23: 492–502. (Reprinted in full in *Midwifery Information and Resource Service Journal (MIDIRS)* (2002) 12: 527–531).

Dykes F (2003) *Infant Feeding Initiative: A Report Evaluating the Breastfeeding Practice Projects 1999–2002*. London: Department of Health.

Dykes F (2005) "Supply" and "Demand": breastfeeding as labour. *Social Science and Medicine* 60 (10): 2283–2293.

Dykes F (2006) *Breastfeeding in Hospital*, Cornwall: Routledge.

Dykes F, Williams C (1999) "Falling by the wayside": a phenomenological exploration of perceived breastmilk inadequacy in lactating women. *Midwifery* 15: 232–246.

Earle S (2002) Why some women do not breastfeed: bottle feeding and father's role. *Midwifery* 16: 323–330.

Ekström A, Widström AM, Nissen E (2005) Process-oriented training in breastfeeding alters attitudes to breastfeeding in health professionals. *Scandinavian Journal of Public Health* 33 (6): 424.

Fewtrell MS (2004) The long term benefits of having been breastfed. *Current Paediatrics* 14: 97–103.

Finigan V, Davies S (2004) 'I just wanted to love, hold him forever': women's lived experience of skin-to-skin contact with their baby immediately after birth. *The Royal College of Midwives. Evidence Based Midwifery Journal* 2 (2): 59–65.

Fishbein M, Ajzen I (1975) *Belief, Attitude, Intention and Behaviour: An Introduction to Theory and Research*, Reading: Addison-Wesley.

Garcia J, Redshaw M, Fitzsimmons B, Keene J (1998) *First Class Delivery: A National Survey of Women's Views of Maternity Care*, Oxon: Audit Commission.

Gerhardt S (2006) *Why Love Matters*. New York, London: Routledge.

Gregg JE (1989) Attitudes of teenagers in Liverpool to breast feeding. *British Medical Journal* 299 (6692): 147–148.

Gross SM, Caulfield LE, Bentley ME (1998) Counselling and motivational video tapes increase duration of breastfeeding in African American WIC participants who initiate breastfeeding. *Journal of the American Dietetic Association* (2): 143–148.

Gwinn ML, Lee NC, Rhodes RH, Layde PM, Rubin GL (1990) Pregnancy, breastfeeding and oral contraceptives and risk of epithelial ovarian cancer. *Journal of Clinical Epidemiology* 43: 559–568.

Hall Moran V, Dinwoodie K, Bramhall R, Dykes F (2000) A critical analysis of the content of tools measuring breastfeeding interactions. *Midwifery* 16: 260–268.

Hamlyn B, Brooker S, Oleinikova K, Wands S (2002) *Infant Feeding Survey 2000*, London: The Stationary Office.

Hartmann PE, Sheriff JL, Kent JC (1995) Maternal nutrition and milk synthesis. *The Proceedings of the Nutrition Society* 54: 379–389.

Hauck FR, Omojokun OO, Siadaty MS (2005) Do pacifiers reduce the risks of SIDS? A meta-analysis. *Pediatrics* 116: 716–723.

Health Development Agency (2003) *The Effectiveness of Public Health Interventions to Promote the Initiation of Breastfeeding: Evidence – Based Briefing*, 1st Edition. Geneva: Health Development Agency, NICE.

Hoddinott P, Pill R (1999) Qualitative study of decisions about infant feeding among women in east end of London. *British Medical Journal* 318: 30–34.

Hoddinott P, Pill R (2000) A qualitative study of women's views about how health professionals communicate about infant feeding. *Health Expectations* 3: 224–233.

Horta BL, Bahl R, Martines JC, Victora CG (2007) *Evidence on the Long Term Effects of Breastfeeding: Systematic Reviews and Meta Analyses*. Geneva: World Health Organization.

Howard CR, Howard FM, Lanphear B, *et al.* (2003) Randomised clinical trial of pacifier use and bottle-feeding or cup-feeding and these effects on breast-feeding. *Pediatrics* 103: e33.

Howie PW, Forsyth JS, Ogston SA, Clark A, Florey C (1990) Protective effect of breastfeeding against infection. *British Journal of Midwifery* 300: 11–16.

Humenick S, Hill P, Spiegelberg R (1998) Breastfeeding and health professionals encouragement. *Journal of Human Lactation* 14: 305–310.

Kisten N, Abrahansan R, Dublin P (1994) Effects of peer counsellors on breast-feeding initiation, exclusivity and duration among low-income urban women. *Journal of Human Lactation* 10: 11–15.

Kramer MS, Chalmers B, Hodnett ED, *et al.* (2001) Promotion of Breastfeeding Intervention Trial (PROBIT) – A randomised trial in the Republic of Belarus. *Journal of American Medical Association* 285: 413–420.

Kroeger M, Smith LJ (2004) *Impact of Birthing Practices on Breastfeeding*, London Barb Mews: Jones and Bartlett Publishers.

Lagercrantz H, Slotkin TA (1986) The stress of being born. *Scientific American* April, 92–102.

Lehtonen J (1998) The effect of nursing on the brain activity of the newborn. *The Journal of Pediatrics* 132: 646–651.

Mahon-Daly P, Andrews GJ (2002) Liminality and breastfeeding: women nego-tiating space and two bodies. *Health and Place* 8: 61–76.

Marild S, Jodal U, Hanson LA (1990) Breastfeeding and urinary tract infection. *Lancet* 336: 942.

Mathur GP, Mathur S, Khanduja GS (1990) Non nutritive suckling and use of pacifiers. *Indian Pediatrics* 27: 1187–1189.

Mattos-Graner RO, de Moraes AB, Rontani RM (2001) Relation of oral yeast infection in Brazilian infants and use of pacifier. *ASDC Journal of Dentistry for Children* 68 (1): 33–36.

McFadden A, Renfrew MJ, Dykes F, Burt S (2006) Addressing the learning needs for breastfeeding: Setting the scene. *Maternal and Child Nutrition* 2: 196–203.

Minchin M (1998) *Artificial Feeding: Risky for any Baby*. Nottingham: La Leche League Books.

Montagu A (1986) *Touching: The Human Significance of the Skin*, 3rd Edition. New York: Harper Row.

Murray SF (1994) *Baby Friendly Mother Friendly*, London: Mosby.

National Case Control Study Group (1993) Breastfeeding and the Risk of breast cancer in young women. United Kingdom National Case Control Study Group. *British Medical Journal* 307: 17–20.

National Institute for Clinical Excellence (2005) *The Effectiveness of Public Health Interventions to Promote the Duration of Breastfeeding [Systematic review]* 1st Edition. London: National Institute for Clinical Excellence.

National Institute for Clinical Excellence (2006a) *Routine Postnatal Care of Women and Their Babies.* Nice Clinical Guideline 37. www.nice.org.uk/CG037.

National Institute for Clinical Excellence (2006b) *Full Guideline 2nd Draft for Consultation Routine Postnatal Care of Women and their Babies.* National Collaborating Centre for Primary Care.

National Institute for Clinical Excellence (2006c) *Effective Action Briefing on the Initiation and Duration of Breastfeeding.* Public Health Collaborating Centre for Maternal and Child Nutrition: Evidence and Guidance. Revised version.

National Institute for Clinical Excellence (2008) *Improving the Nutrition of Pregnant and Breastfeeding Mothers and Children in Low-income Households. NICE Public Health Guidance 11.* London: National Institute for Clinical Excellence.

Newcombe PA, Storer BE, Longneckr MP (1994) Lactation and a reduced risk of premenopausal breast cancer. *The New England Journal of Medicine* 330: 81–87.

Nicoll A, Thayaparan B, Newell M, Rundall P (2002) Breast feeding policy, promotion and practice in Europe. Results of a survey with non-governmental organizations. *Journal of Nutritional and Environmental Medicine* 12 (3): 255–264.

North West Framework for Action (2008) *Addressing Health Inequalities A North West Breastfeeding Framework for Action*, Manchester: North West Regional Public Health Group.

Odent M (2003) *Birth and Breastfeeding*, Sussex: Clairview Books.

Palmer G (2003) It's the belief that's important. *Practising Midwife* 6 (10): 20–22.

Paronen J, Knip M, Savilahti E (2000) Effect of cow's milk exposure and maternal type 1 diabetes on cellular and humoral immunization to dietary insulin in infants at genetic risk for type 1 diabetes. Finnish trial to reduce IDDM in the Genetically at Risk Study. *Diabetes* 49: 1657–1665.

Penrose–Arlotti J, Hanson-Cottrell B, Hughes-Lee S, Curtin JJ (1998) Breastfeeding among low income women with and without peer support. *Journal of Community Health Nursing* 15 (3): 163–178.

Perez-Escamillia R, Pollitt E, Lonnerdal B, Dewey KG (1994) Infant feeding policies in maternity wards and their effect on breastfedding success: an analytical overview. *American Journal of Public Health* 84(1): 89–97.

Pettitt DJ, Bennett PH, Saad MF, Charles MD (1997) Abnormal glucose tolerance during pregnancy in Pima Indian Women: Long term effects on offspring. *Lancet* 350 (9072): 166–168.

Philipp BL, Malone KL, Cimo S, Merewood A (2003) Sustained breastfeeding rates at a US Baby-Friendly Hospital. *Pediatrics* 112: e234–e236.

Porteous RM, Kaufman K, Rush J (2000) The effect of individualised professional support on duration of breastfeeding: a randomised control trial. *Journal of Human Lactation* 16 (4): 303–308.

Renfrew MJ, Dyson L, Wallace L, D'Souza L, McCormick FM, Spiby H (2005) *The Effectiveness of Health Interventions to Promote the Duration of Breastfeeding; Systematic Review*, London: National Institute for Health and Clinical Excellence.

Righard L, Alade MO (1990) The time has come to reassess delivery ward routines. *Lancet* 336: 1105–1107.

Riordan J (2005) *Breastfeeding and Human Lactation*, 3rd Edition. Library of Congress Cataloguing-in-Publication Sudbury, MA: Jones & Bartlett Publishers.

Robertson A, Minkler M (1994) New Health Promotion Movement: a critical examination. *Health Education Quarterly* 21 (3): 295–312.

Rogers C (1961) *On Becoming a Person*, Boston: Houghton Miltin.

Rossenblatt KA, Thomas DB (1993) WHO collaborative study of neoplasia and steroid contraceptives. *International Journal of Epidemiology* 22: 192–197.

Scott JA, Binns CW (1999) Factors associated with the initiation and duration of breastfeeding. *Breastfeeding Review* 71: 15–16.

Shore C, Burrs S, Elliot K, Harper M, Jones S, McMahon J, Owen K, Radford A, Williams A (1998) *Breastfeeding in Paediatric Units; Guidance for Good Practice*. London: RCN.

Short RV (1994) What the breast does for the baby, and what the baby does for the breast. *Aust NZ Journal Obstet Gynaecol* 34 (3): 262–264.

Simmons V (2003) Inconsistent advice and practice:part 3. *British Journal of Midwifery* 11: 564–567.

Sirkoski J, Renfrew MJ (1999) *Support for breastfeeding mothers (Cochrane Review)*. In *The Cochrane Library*, Issue 2, Oxford Update Software.

Smale M, Renfrew MJ, Marshall JL, Spiby H (2006) Turning policy into practice; more difficult than it seems. The case of breastfeeding education. *Maternal and Child Nutrition* 2: 103–113.

Tappin D (1997) Health Service potential cost savings with increased breastfeeding rates. *Greater Glasgow Health Board Breastfeeding Strategy*, Yorkhill: Peach Unit

Tarkka MT, Paunonen M, Laippala P (1998) What contributes to breastfeeding success after childbirth in a maternity ward in Finland? *Birth* 25: 175–181.

UK National Case Control Study Group (1993) Breastfeeding and the risks of breast cancer in young women. *British Medical Journal* 307: 17–20.

UNICEF (1991) *State of Worlds Children*, Oxford: Oxford University Press.

UNICEF (2007) http://www.babyfriendly.org.uk/.

UNICEF (2008) *Infant Feeding Survey 2005: Findings Related to the Baby Friendly Initiative*. http://ic.nhs.uk/statistics-and-data-collections/health-and-lifestyles/infant-feeding/infant-feeding-survey-2005.

UNICEF UK BFI (1998) *A Seven Point Plan for the Protection; Promotion and Support of Breastfeeding in Community Health Care Settings*. London: UNICEF. http://www.babyfriendly.org.uk/.

UNICEF UK BFI (2005) Baby Friendly Initiative Teaching Packs. Available at: http://www.babyfriendly.org.uk/teaching-packs.asp (accessed 11/11/2008).

Valdes V, Pugin E, Miriam H, *et al.* (1995) The effects on professional practice of a three day course on breastfeeding. *Journal of Human Lactation* 11: 185–190.

Vogel AM, Mitchell EA (1998) The establishment and duration of breastfeeding, part 1: hospital influences. *Breastfeeding Review* 6: 5–9.

Whelan A, Lupton P (1998) Promoting successful breastfeeding among women of low income. *Midwifery* 14: 94–100.

Wiberg B, Humble K, de Chateau P (1989) Long-term effect on mother-infant behaviour of extra contact during the first hour postpartum: follow-up at three years. *Scandinavian Journal of Social Medicine* 17: 181–191.

Wilson AC, Forsyth JS, Greene SA, Irvine L, Hay C, Howie EW (1998) Relation of infant diet to childhood health: seven year follow up of cohort of children in Dundee infant feeding study. *British Medical Journal* 316: 21–25.

Woolridge M (1994) The baby friendly hospital initiative UK. *Modern Midwife* 4 (50): 29–30.

World Health Organisation (1981) *International Code of Marketing of Breast-Milk Substitutes*. Geneva: WHO.

World Health Organisation (1998) *Evidence for the Ten Steps To Successful Breast-feeding*, Geneva: WHO.

World Health Organisation (2007) *Evidence on the Long-Term Effects of Breastfeeding: Systematic Reviews and Meta-analyses*. Geneva: Department of Child and Adolescent Health and Development (CAH), World Health Organization.

Wright S (1998) Politicisation of "culture." *Anthropology in Action* 5: 3–10.

Chapter 8
Engaging Vulnerable Women and Families: Postnatal Care

Anita Fleming and Jill Cooper

> It is easy to be intolerant and fail to understand the complexities of living in poverty. Women are individual and have individual needs – Midwives must look beyond their own prejudices and the stereotypes peddled in the media. Most women are just trying to get through in their own way, they love their kids and do their best, and from the midwives they don't want judgements, labels – all they want is 'a bit of respect'.
>
> (Hunt 2009, Personal communications)

Introduction

Current drivers for maternity services are directing commissioners and service providers to explore innovative ways of engaging with vulnerable women and families (DoH 2007; Darzi 2008) to address health inequalities and influence the health and well-being of future generations. Pregnancy and the first 3 years of life are vital to child development, life chances and future achievement, and midwives are ideally placed to identify children and families at risk and to signpost families to extensive support. Postnatal care is one of the most important aspects of maternity care, but has previously suffered from a lack of attention and resources (Bick 2008). Many current maternity service models do not acknowledge the fact that postnatal care is an essential link in the continuum of maternity care, and potentially the foundation of future child and maternal health, especially for those most vulnerable.

But what is meant by vulnerable? Are the needs of these families really any different to others, and does targeted or directed support influence outcomes? What effect does poverty have on women and families, and can midwives make a difference? This chapter will consider these questions and propose ideas as to how the needs of all women might be addressed, with particular regard to those women and families deemed most vulnerable, during the postnatal period.

Vulnerability – by whose definition?

The Oxford English Dictionary (2008) defines vulnerable as 'that may be wounded; susceptible of receiving wounds or physical injury'. However, in this instance it may be thought that vulnerability may arise as a result of physical, emotional or environmental factors and not simply result in a physical injury. Families living in poverty in inner city or rural areas may be seen as vulnerable, but the family living in relative monetary affluence totally isolated from family, friends and others may also face consequences from isolation.

Generally speaking, the main drivers of maternity services in recent years use the word 'vulnerable' when referring to women or families where there is evidence to show that these groups experience poorer obstetric and neonatal outcomes (DoH 2007; Lewis 2007; CEMACH 2008). The latest Confidential Enquiry into Maternal and Child Health (CEMACH) report (Lewis 2007) makes the statement that 'the link between adverse pregnancy outcomes and vulnerability and social exclusion are never more starkly demonstrated than by this Enquiry'. However, Lavender *et al.* (2007) raised the issue that little is known of the evidential link between inadequate antenatal care and perinatal and maternal outcome, and undertook a structured review to pursue the matter further. The findings demonstrate a lack of both quantitative and qualitative UK research, which addresses the phenomenon of late antenatal attendance or non-attendance, though the qualitative review does provide some understanding of why women fail to access antenatal care, including factors such as pregnancy rejection/acceptance, and personal capacity or incapacity to act. The review also suggests that continuing access for women in high-risk and marginalised groups appears to depend on a strategy referred to as 'weighing up and balancing out' of the perceived gains and losses of attendance to them and their babies. The recommendation from the review is that more prospective, UK-based studies are required to explore further what works in improving access for disadvantaged groups, and whether improved access improves outcomes.

An important, fundamental factor that must be taken into account when working with women who perhaps need more support owing to any vulnerability is that they do not want to be singled out, or made to feel different, whether that be being judged or segregated and patronised. The evidence is clear that inequalities in health exist and that those families living with any vulnerability are more likely to suffer poorer health outcomes. In her study of women living in poverty, Hunt (2004) warns health professionals and leaders not to simply place women in categories, which could in turn perpetuate adverse outcomes.

Who are 'vulnerable' women and what are the issues and consequences?

Bostock (2003) defines inequalities in health as the difference in morbidity and mortality between individuals of higher or lower socio-economic status, to the extent that the differences are perceived to be unfair. A complex network of factors contribute to this inequality with determinants such as income, education, employment, environment and lifestyle behaviours such as smoking, drinking, diet and risk-taking having an impact on ill health (DoH 1998). We have explored some of the areas of vulnerability for women and families, presenting reasons for poor outcomes and useful interventions. Whilst we acknowledge that women are 'grouped' within the literature, there is a sense that by doing so, we are placing them in structural categories, and therefore marginalising them even further. In addition, it must be remembered that some women may fall into more than one 'group', or are part of all groups, and their complex lives are placing them on the very edge of life itself. Some women have multiple indicators for poorer health outcomes, for example, if they smoke, and have mental health issues, and live in an area of extreme social deprivation. Each factor interrelates with the other: the environment they live in may impact on their mental health, and smoking may be viewed as a solitary 'pleasure' within the complexity. However, women may be deemed vulnerable due to their social status or place of residence, and there is a tendency by some healthcare professionals to 'judge' women by these standards, even if the women have made individual positive life choices for themselves and their families.

Poverty and social disadvantage

In their research into postnatal care, Bick & MacArthur (1995) found that childbirth makes some women ill, and it is more likely to make them ill if they are poor. Low income is a problem that a substantial proportion of childbearing women face in the United Kingdom, with one in every four children living in a household with below half average income (Rowe *et al.* 2003). This is more likely in families where one or more parent is out of work, in lone parent families, in ethnic minority families and in families with a disabled member. Owing to the lack of appropriate data, it is not possible to make a direct link between low income and poor outcomes of pregnancy, but there is a wealth of data that points to worse outcomes and poorer ongoing health for babies, children and mothers in lower socio-economic groups or living in areas of social deprivation compared with more affluent families. The place a person lives in, or environmental circumstances, can influence their level of exposure to health risks by limiting the chances and opportunities they have to make healthy lifestyle choices DoH (2003). When considering maternal and perinatal health outcomes and the link between social factors and poor outcomes, the Index of Multiple Deprivation (IMD) is frequently used. This is a ward-based measure with seven sub-domains (income, employment, health, education, housing and services, environment and crime). Larger values indicate higher degrees of deprivation.

The Joseph Rowntree Foundation (1999) described the effect that poverty and debt have on psychological health, and linked low income with an increase in stress, depression and social isolation. Health services are less likely to be accessed by those living in disadvantaged areas, and it has been suggested that inhibiting factors may be lack of social networks, lack of role models, lack of confidence in service providers, and also inflexible working patterns. Consequently, families in these communities may access health services in different or less appropriate ways, for example, using emergency services rather than preventative ones (DoH 2005).

The consequences of these factors are highlighted in the Perinatal Mortality 2006 report (CEMACH 2008), with over a third of all stillbirths and neonatal deaths being born to mothers living in the most deprived areas. In addition, compared to rates in the least deprived area, those resident in the most deprived area had a twofold increase in stillbirth and neonatal mortality rates. There has been no improvement in the rates since 2000, and other demographic factors known to be associated with stillbirths such as obesity, ethnicity, deprivation and maternal age may be contributing to this lack of progress. Maternal mortality rates from 2003 to 2005 similarly demonstrated rates in the most deprived areas being around five times higher than in the least deprived.

Smoking

Smoking in pregnancy is recognised as a key determinant of low birth weight and is also closely linked to socio-economic status (Babb *et al.* 2004), with the percentage of singleton births with low birth weights being higher for babies with mothers residing in the more deprived areas. Babies born to mothers who smoke are twice as likely to have low birth weights than those born to non-smokers (Bull *et al.* 2003), and these infants also have almost five times the risk of sudden infant death than those born to women who do not smoke (Richardson

2001). Smoking was also found to be a factor associated with increased maternal mortality rates (Lewis 2007).

Breastfeeding

Hamlyn *et al.* (2002) demonstrated the fact that women from dis-advantaged communities or of lower socio-economic status are less likely to breastfeed their babies. Chapter 7 eloquently highlights the issues pertaining to health inequalities and breastfeeding, and proposes evidence-based interventions to attempt to reverse the trend. Midwives and peer support workers should be aware of the potential conse-quence of reduced breastfeeding rates amongst some populations, that is, poorer health outcomes for mothers and babies. Community models of breastfeeding support, that is, mother to mother or peer support, offer a twofold opportunity to improve health and well-being through improved breastfeeding. When community women and mothers are empowered through learning new skills, there is increased capacity in breastfeeding support at a local level that is not dependant on health professionals, whose episodes of ability to assist is time limited. Chapter 5 offers an insight into community models of support, outlin-ing the processes and benefits, and uses examples to demonstrate the potential impact.

Complex social issues and child protection

The review of maternal deaths (Lewis 2007) identified that the women with socially complex pregnancies were often known to social services, particularly child protection services, and that these women were particularly vulnerable. Many hid the pregnancy from social services and avoided maternity care even though they were at increased risk of medical or mental health problems, and the stresses of child protection conferences and the removal of babies into care further compounded the risks. During the 3-year period, 41 women died following a child protection care conference, 34 of whom were misusers of substances. Twenty-three women died after their babies had been removed into care – 5 from suicide and 18 from substance misuse, which could not be disproved as intentional acts. While it is acknowledged that child protection is of the utmost importance, care and support for the mother during such a distressing time is also paramount (Lewis 2007).

Midwives in the United Kingdom will be increasingly familiar with the Common Assessment Framework (CAF), which is a response to child protection issues that helps practitioners assess children's additional needs for services earlier and more effectively, develop a common understanding of those needs, and agree on a process for working together to meet them. The aim of the CAF is to provide better services earlier, and without the need for the family to repeat their story for a number of different, overlapping assessments. As such, early common assessment is part of the government's strategy to shift the focus from dealing with the consequences of difficulties in children's lives to preventing things from going wrong in the first place. Some common assessments will result in the identification of a lead professional (who may be the midwife) who will coordinate the actions set out in the assessment (CO 2006).

Ethnicity/migrant women

Stillbirth and neonatal mortality rates are significantly higher for Black and Asian ethnic groups (Lewis 2007), in addition to maternal mortality rates for Black African women (including newly arrived refugees and asylum seekers) being almost six times higher than for White ethnic women (Lewis 2007).

The increasing numbers of migrant women seeking maternity care in the United Kingdom often have poorer general health, more complicated pregnancies and obstetric histories, and may have significant underlying medical conditions. Women seeking asylum are often grouped together in accommodation. A number of professionals and women, consulted for a Needs Assessment conducted by Brunel University, commented that the main source of support for Unaccompanied Asylum Seeking Children (UASC) was their peers. Although in many ways this is very positive, these young pregnant women and mothers were excluded from accurate information and knowledge shared from other more experienced women. Where young women are grouped together in accommodation they can become insular, which may lead to perpetuating poor or inadequate information (Gaudion & Allotey 2008).

In other areas, schemes which specifically target lone mothers, those newly arrived in the United Kingdom, have been set up in order to ensure these women are getting the support they need. This group is likely to be disadvantaged when accessing care due to lack of knowledge of availability and also language difficulties.

Teenage pregnancy

Teenage parenthood is perceived to be both a cause and a consequence of social exclusion (Hollings *et al.* 2007). The Social Exclusion Unit (SEU) (1999) found that teenage parents are more likely to be unemployed, live in poverty, give birth to low birth weight babies, who are likely to be at increased risk of childhood accidents as toddlers. The significance of this link with social exclusion is that teenage parents therefore are themselves more likely to be in poorer health, with reduced access to health and social support, resulting in poorer health outcomes for themselves and their babies (Swann *et al.* 2003).

Mothers aged less than 20 years were the age group with the most neonatal deaths, and one of the age groups with the highest rates of stillbirth (Lewis 2007).

Alcohol and substance misuse

Both medical and social adverse effects of substance misuse in pregnancy are well-documented. Hepburn (2005) discovered a higher incidence of preterm birth, low birth weight babies, and sudden infant deaths among pregnant drug users. Consideration must also be given to the fact that women who misuse drugs and alcohol may be doubly vulnerable if they are already marginalised through poverty or coming from a disadvantaged background, and may have low levels of literacy and numeracy as a result of lack of education and employment.

These women often have chaotic lifestyles and complex needs. In order to fund a drug or excessive alcohol habit, women often find themselves in danger by becoming victims of sexual exploitation, which increases the risk of physical and psychological danger, blood-borne viruses, degradation and potential drug-related death (McIver 2007).

The review of maternal deaths between 2003 and 2005 identified substance misuse as being associated, either directly or indirectly, with the deaths of 57 women (Lewis 2007).

Perinatal mental health

Perinatal mental health problems are common: many are serious and they can have long-lasting effects on maternal health and child development. Chapter 4 describes the effect of motherhood in terms on emotional influence and changes in mood. Postnatal depression (PND) is a recognised and treatable illness that affects approximately 10–15% of mothers and 10% of fathers. It may come on immediately after the arrival of the baby but can also present later, or go unrecognised for weeks or months.

Psychiatric disorder, both in the antenatal period and following the birth, is not uncommon. These may be new episodes or recurrences of pre-existing conditions (Lewis 2007). Ten percent of new mothers are likely to develop a depressive illness in the year following the birth of their baby (O'Hara & Swain 1996), with between a third and a half of these suffering from a severe depressive illness (Cox *et al.* 1993). During this time, at least 2% of new mothers will be referred to a psychiatric team, and four women per thousand will require admission to a psychiatric unit, of whom two per thousand will have puerperal psychosis (Oates 1996).

Most women who have mental health problems either during pregnancy or following birth will experience mild depressive illness, often accompanied with anxiety. These are of equal prevalence in the antenatal period and after birth, and probably no more common than at other times (O'Hara & Swain 1996). However, where the risk of developing a serious mental illness, such as bipolar disorder or severe depressive illness, is reduced during pregnancy, it is significantly increased following the birth, particularly in the first 3 months (Kendell *et al.* 1987).

Women who have suffered from a serious mental illness in the past, either after the birth of a baby or at other times, have a higher risk of developing a post-partum onset illness even if they have been well during the pregnancy and for a long time before – the risk is at least one in two (Wieck *et al.* 1991; Robertson *et al.* 2005). There is also evidence that a woman with a family history of bipolar disorder has an increased risk of developing puerperal psychosis following childbirth (Robertson *et al.* 2005). It is important to remember that the review of maternal deaths between 2003 and 2005 reported 33 deaths from suicide (Lewis 2007).

Traumatic birth and post-traumatic stress

PND and puerperal psychosis are conditions that are now much better understood and accepted by the public, but there is not the same understanding regarding issues associated with post-traumatic stress and childbirth (Dearman *et al.* 2007).

National Institute for Health and Clinical Excellence (NICE) (2005) recognised childbirth as a significant stressor that can place some women at risk of developing the full range of post-traumatic stress disorder (PTSD). Factors including unexpected Caesarean section, prolonged labour with inadequate pain relief and hostile staff have been identified as possibly predisposing women to develop PTSD (Ryding *et al.* 1998). Dearman *et al.* (2007) reported the prevalence of PTSD following childbirth to be between 2 and 7%.

Symptoms are not always recognised and may be confused with PND (Beech & Robinson 1985), and if untreated, may develop into enduring health problems (Beck 2004).

A combination of objective and subjective factors, including mode of birth and feelings of loss of control and dignity, have been used to describe PTSD and childbirth (Beck 2004), with women using language more often associated with victims of torture or rape to describe their birth experiences (Dearman *et al.* 2007).

Domestic abuse

The Department of Health (2006) defines domestic abuse as

> Any incident of threatening behaviour, abuse or abuse (psychological, physical, sexual, financial or emotional) between adults who are or have been intimate partners or family members, regardless of gender or sexuality.
>
> (DoH 2006)

Domestic abuse is a serious, but sadly often overlooked, cause of maternal and infant morbidity and mortality (Drife and Lewis 1998). It often remains hidden and undisclosed, making it difficult to discover the exact prevalence (Price 2007). However, there is evidence to show that male violence in the home may be triggered or exacerbated during pregnancy, instead of it being a time of peace and safety (Royal College of Midwives 1999). It is known that 30% of cases of domestic abuse first start during pregnancy, and that 40–60% of women who have experienced domestic abuse are then abused during the pregnancy. Very worryingly, more than 14% of maternal deaths occur in women who have told a health professional that they are in an abusive relationship (DoH 2006). In the review of maternal deaths between 2003 and 2005 (Lewis 2007), 70 women died who had features of domestic abuse and this abuse proved to be fatal for the 19 women who were murdered.

The above-named groups do not form an exhaustive list of those deemed to be vulnerable, but they are examples of where there is evidence to demonstrate the need for targeted service provision to try to improve the adverse outcomes identified. Indeed, for many women, all the above factors feature at some point in their lives, and in some communities the percentage of women living with multiple complex social problems is significant. The Government and the Department of Health in the United Kingdom have prioritised the reduction of health inequalities within maternity services and early years, through various specific policy drivers, (DoH/DES 2004; CO 2006) specific resource allocation for projects and developments. One such project is the 'Family Nurse Partnership (FNP) Programme' that is designed to specifically meet the needs of young first-time mothers and is based on a similar programme developed in the United States (DCSF 2008a). FNP has three primary aims:

- To improve pregnancy outcomes
- To improve child health
- To improve parents' economic self-sufficiency

The programme was initiated in the United States and three large-scale randomised controlled trials have shown many benefits for the new

Table 8.1 Key risk and protective factors during pregnancy and up to the age of 2 for negative outcomes in later life.

	Risk factors	*Protective factors*
Pregnancy	Prematurity/birth factors	Genetic predisposition
	Obstetric difficulties	Having someone to confide in
	Genetic predisposition	
	Stress in pregnancy	
	Teenage pregnancy	
	Smoking in pregnancy	
	Neglected neighbourhood	
	Low income	
	Poor housing	
Age 0–2	Impaired attachment	Resilience
	Infant's temperament	Strong attachment to at least one carer
	ADHD-hyperactivity	Bonding with child
	Postnatal depression	
	Harsh parenting style	
	Rejection	
	Hitting/frequent smacking	
	Low-level stimulation	
	Socio-economic stress	

ADHD, attention deficit hyperactivity disorder.
Adapted from Sutton et al. (2004) ibid. Factors listed relate to risk of committing crime and anti-social behaviour. In Cabinet Office (2006) Reaching out: an action plan on social exclusion HMSO.

family, based not only on health improvements, but also on increased employment levels and fewer, more spaced out subsequent pregnancies. Regular visits by a known and trusted carer often mean that other services can become involved and provide further support when needed.

UK policy recommends a model of care for midwives and health visitors based on 'progressive universalism' from pregnancy until the age of 2, where there is intensive support for those at risk and a lighter touch for others (CO 2006). In some areas, commissioners have worked with maternity services, and helped to develop such models, through specialised commissioned services. The Cabinet Office (2006) developed an action plan to tackle social exclusion and utilised evidence of effective interventions in their proposals (see Table 8.1).

Universal postnatal care, midwives and maternity care workers

Owing to the provision of a universally available maternity service in the United Kingdom, midwives are in a perfect position to offer guidance to vulnerable families, at a time when parents may be highly receptive to external advice and support. National Institute for Health and Clinical Excellence (NICE) guidance on routine postnatal care suggests that planning should begin in the antenatal period (NICE 2006). However, a lack of time spent preparing for the postnatal period means that women are arriving on postnatal wards not knowing what to expect, and are therefore unprepared for the impact of birth on their physical and emotional health (Beake *et al.* 2005). In addition to this, because of limited provision of resources, UK midwives are under pressure to discharge women home quickly from postnatal wards, and limits are being placed on the number of postnatal home visits (Bick 2008). If support is limited for all women, there is increased risk of those most vulnerable to becoming even more marginalised, with some potential for consequences described earlier.

When providing routine postnatal care, midwives and maternity support workers should aim to see the new mother not only as an individual, but also as part of a wider network, whether that be a positive or a negative one. This will help carers to determine what support she needs, where to signpost, and what priorities need to be considered when helping her to make appropriate choices. When postnatal care is under-resourced and time for women is limited, these simple strategies will maximise the potential for the provision of support and enhance opportunities for promoting confidence in women's ability to nurture and parent their children.

For these strategies to be successful, midwives and other maternity care workers should reflect on their own internal prejudices in relation to class structures and socio-cultural beliefs. When considering the effect of poverty on women, Hunt (2004) stated that not only does poverty have a detrimental effect on women's mental and physical health but it also appears to influence the quality of care that some women receive from some midwives.

It is worth remembering a basic recommendation from the NICE Postnatal Care Guideline (NICE 2006):

> Women and their families should always be treated with kindness, respect and dignity. The views, beliefs and values of the woman, her partner and her family in relation to her care and that of her baby should be sought and respected at all times.

Children's centres

Children's centres provide multi-agency services that are flexible and meet the needs of young children and their families. The core offer includes integrated early learning, care, family support, health services, outreach services to children and families not attending the centre and access to training and employment advice. Each centre aims to provide high-quality learning and full day care for children from birth (DCSF 2008b).

It is proposed that by 2010 every community will be served by a children's centre, ensuring that every child has the opportunity of having the best start in life. These services will be permanent and universal, and though they will vary according to the local needs of that particular community, they will generally include services such as integrated early education and childcare; support for parents and families; child and family health services, including antenatal and postnatal care and breastfeeding support and helping parents into work (DCSF 2008b).

Recent years have seen an increase in the variety of maternity services being delivered in children's centres. They have proved to be popular venues for antenatal education sessions and drop-ins, as well as for antenatal clinics where the trend has been to move out of GP clinics and health centres into the often more accessible children's centres, which provides an invaluable opportunity for the centres to promote their service to parents and parents-to-be in the area (Slater & Byrom 2006). One single, yet crucial, benefit for delivering services from children's centres is that women and families are introduced to other (social and educational) support available for them and their children.

With recommendations being made in documents such as Maternity Matters (DoH 2007) for maternity services to offer a 'choice of place of postnatal care' children's centres provide ideal venues with the scope to develop new, innovative ways of delivering postnatal services.

Targeted support

Since 1999, public health targeted approaches to maternity services have developed and continue to expand in the United Kingdom. Several proposed interventions are discussed in this section; some based on research evidence and some suggested good practice points. It must be acknowledged, however, that although targeted support for some women is essential, midwives and maternity care workers need to consider the effect of their individual attitudes to poverty and indifference, as a potential reason for women's reluctance to engage with health services. In addition, the mobilisation of other agencies in providing support is crucial, and is detailed in Chapter 9.

Ensuring that antenatal care is accessed and viewed by women as a worthwhile experience maximises potential for access to postnatal care. If a woman has been able to build up a trusting relationship with her caregivers during her pregnancy, the door is opened for her to continue through to postnatal care too.

'Sure Start' local programmes set out to improve health and social outcomes for children, bringing together early education, child care and health (www.surestart.gov.uk/), from pre-birth to school age. Within the last decade, 'Sure Start' provided one of the first opportunities for midwives to work with other agencies during pregnancy and the postnatal period. In addition, schemes that provide continuity of caregiver for vulnerable women such as the Albany Practice (Huber & Sandall 2006), Blackburn with Darwen Midwifery Caseload Practice, and other caseloading models are not only appreciated by women and midwives, but also result in increased uptake of both antenatal and postnatal care, increased breastfeeding rates, and reduced low birth weight (Fleming 2008). Providing one-to-one care throughout their childbearing experience places women firmly in the centre of their care, promoting opportunity for increased self-esteem and positive birth outcomes. The Blackburn with Darwen Midwifery Group Practice (BwDMGP) was established in 2004 to provide one-to-one care to all women within a defined geographical 'Sure Start' area (Byrom & Downe 2007). In 2006, the decision was taken to broaden the geographical area, and to limit referral to those women deemed most vulnerable in an attempt to improve maternal and infant health outcomes. The referral criteria includes the following:

- Women under the care of the **community mental health team (CMHT)**
- Women with **complex** child protection issues
- Women who are **HIV positive**
- Women with fetal abnormalities with a **poor prognosis**
- **Unsupported** asylum seekers

Also,

- Women having had a previous traumatic birth or with severe anxiety about birth. Women who abuse drugs or alcohol – also **referred to Drugs Liaison Midwife**
- Teenagers under the age of 16 – **referred first to Teenage Pregnancy midwife**
- Other women with an **identified need** for one-to-one care.

Within Blackburn with Darwen, a triangle of need has helped to shape midwifery care provision and the development of a service that best meets the needs of those women accessing the service (Figure 8.1).

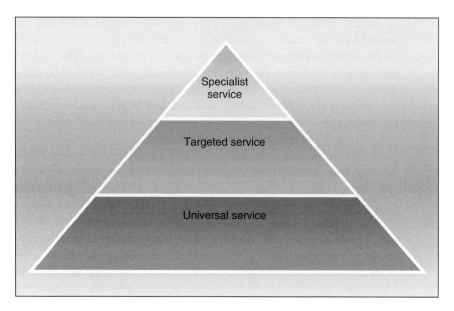

Figure 8.1 Triangle of need/support service.

The following story from a midwife working with the BwDMGP demonstrates the value of extra support and guidance during the antenatal period subsequently having an impact in the postnatal period.

Case study 1

I first met Saira at the beginning of her first pregnancy. She was in her early 20s, living alone in a hostel and had a partner who dropped in now and again. Saira had stopped seeing her family who lived in a nearby town because she was worried about them knowing she was pregnant as they didn't approve of her partner. Saira was assigned to the caseload team for one-to-one midwifery care and I became her named midwife.

Throughout her pregnancy we got to know each other. I arranged for Saira to get extra support through a family support worker from her nearby children's centre, and with their help she moved into her own house. Gradually Saira began to trust me and I began to understand her fears and worries. We spent time thinking and talking about the birth, but more importantly about being a mum, and above all I listened. It was important that Saira thought about her own support needs as she looked into the future. With her support worker Saira started making her own preparations for the coming birth and for caring for the baby.

Saira had a quick and straightforward labour and birth and was soon home with her son Ali. She instinctively knew how to care for him best, as she was realising her own abilities – she had laboured well and now she would mother well too. Saira had chosen to breastfeed and joined a local breastfeeding support group, where she won an award for her dedication to breastfeeding and her support for others. Saira tentatively contacted one of her brothers and slowly but surely began to first talk by phone, and then face to face with her mum, finally going to visit, taking her son with her, much to her mum's delight.

At our last visit, we spent some time reflecting on our journey together and I reminded Saira of the first time we had met and how anxious and nervous she had been. In front of me was a relaxed, confident young woman who said 'Well, I have to put Ali first now, I have to get it right for him'.

For Saira, becoming a mother had also been a journey to find her own strength. By receiving care from people she knew and had a great deal of trust in, she was able to explore her own challenges, knowing that there were people there to help if needed. As a midwife, knowing what other support was available for Saira meant that we could all work together as she met the challenges she faced.

Meeting the needs of pregnant women seeking asylum

McLeish (2005) described the hostility and racism experienced by women accessing maternity services in England, leading to their feeling valueless and hardly likely to access postnatal care. Asylum seekers are often moved to different towns and cities during their pregnancies, which is not conducive to establishing a support network and which can be particularly stressful for single women. Some areas have developed support and befriending schemes, which aim to help these women integrate into the local community with help for other asylum seekers who have been in the area longer. Leeds Asylum Seekers Support Network (LASSN) matches volunteers one-to-one with a client – pregnant women, new mothers and mothers of young children are a priority (LASSN 2008). The aim of the scheme is to offer befriending, orientation and companionship and ensure that appropriate health services are accessed. A Mother and Baby Group also encourages women to interact with local health professionals such as midwives and nurses who lead discussions on pregnancy, birth and early motherhood.

Again, by developing relationships in the antenatal period, longer term health benefits provided by continuing interaction with services are likely and ignoring the needs of pregnant asylum seekers and their babies is short-sighted (McLeish 2002). See Chapter 9 for more examples of good practice.

Providing services tailor-made to suit the women and their situation pays dividends. In Bristol, a bilingual outreach worker has been employed to work with health visitors when visiting women from the Somali community. The women trust the outreach worker, who is from the same background as themselves (and so understands the horrors they may have witnessed in Somalia) and can put their fears and concerns into context and provides an invaluable link into the healthcare system (White 2007).

Perinatal mental health support

CEMACH (2004) made recommendations with regard to midwifery practice and maternal mental health, which included the need for midwives to ask specific questions at booking regarding any previous episodes of mental illness in a systematic but sensitive way, and that women identified to have a history of long and enduring or severe mental health problems should be referred to a psychiatrist with a view to agreeing on a management plan, because of the risks of recurrence. Dearman *et al.* (2007) described how following the booking visit, midwives can subsequently support women through the process of referral to psychiatric services and work in partnership with them to agree on a management plan.

Some areas have developed successful perinatal mental health services, in line with recommendations from NICE (2007), and there are various voluntary and charitable organisations[1], which offer guidance and support for women and partners suffering from this condition. Chapter 4 provides some description of the emotional aspects of motherhood, and how this impacts physiologically.

Domestic abuse: what can midwives do?

In the first instance, midwives need the resources and training to deliver routine enquiry to women in contact with maternity services, (DoH 2000, 2005). The Department of Health in the United Kingdom has developed a useful resource for health professionals to assist with understanding and supporting domestic abuse (DoH 2005). As health professionals supporting those who are experiencing domestic abuse, it is important to understand and accept that sometimes women will make decisions that others find hard to understand (DoH 2005). Overcoming the frustrations and misperceptions forms an important part of providing support. Domestic abuse is always the responsibility of the perpetrator; it is inappropriate to blame the abused woman – it is not her fault (DoH 2005). For a lot of women coping with domestic abuse, speaking to somebody about it and finding ways to create a safer life can take a long time. It is a long process – not a single event, and therefore it is important to continue to support them. It is important to remember that there may be child protection concerns within the abuse, either in relation to the unborn baby or other children in the family.

The Department of Health resource mentioned above (2005) advocates certain measures for healthcare workers in terms of support as follows:

- Focus on the woman's safety and that of her children, if she has any.
- Give her information and refer her to relevant agencies.
- Make it easy for a woman to talk about her experiences.
- Support and reassure her.
- Be non-judgmental.

Support for teenagers and women who misuse drugs

Many maternity services have developed specialist support midwifery posts to provide extra care for women in these categories. The midwives may see women as part of their caseload or provide additional support to the woman's midwifery team. Where these posts are not established, midwives and maternity workers should be fully aware of the potential special needs for the woman and her baby and be knowledgeable of the support mechanisms available to appropriately signpost. Many maternity services have employed teenage pregnancy midwives, who provide extra support and assistance to teenage parents. In a report (DoH/DfES 2007) highlighting what teenagers feel about maternity and health visiting services, young mothers felt that maternity services were unresponsive to their particular needs and that sometimes midwives and other maternity staff were judgemental, which put them off attending antenatal classes. Those who had experienced a specialist teenage pregnancy service welcomed the provision of dedicated services for young mothers – rather than all-age services (DoH/DfES 2007).

For women who misuse drugs, multidisciplinary care is necessary to optimise outcomes, because the financial, psychological, social and domestic problems associated with drug misuse are often of greater importance than the physical and medical concerns (Prentice 2007). Specialist midwifery posts enable the coordination of appropriate care and support between acute hospital trusts, community midwives, general practitioners, mental health and drug services, social services and sometimes the police.

Engaging women from black and minority ethnic groups

Lack of a common language, no understanding of British culture and medical care and fear of living in a new environment can all be factors for women not seeking appropriate care, or feeling reluctant to engage with health services. Midwives and support workers have developed innovative ways of engaging women from minority groups, using simple strategies such as changing times of appointments to coincide with cultural or religious traditions to enhance participation in care.

Projects have been developed in many areas, which aim to reverse this and encourage women to take an important role in their care. In Birmingham, Gateway Family Services support women by using Pregnancy Outreach workers who offer emotional and practical support through pregnancy, birth and parenting, using an appropriate language, which the woman understands (Gateway Family Services 2008). This support includes working with midwives to ensure that women access services and also maintaining links with the community to lessen isolation.

It is important that midwives do not use family members to translate during consultations or contact, as women may feel embarrassed or inhibited to answer questions honestly, especially in relation to mental health issues or domestic abuse. The use of interpreters and advocacy workers is essential when providing services for this community, but when this is not possible the use of national interpreting support lines such as Language Line[2] is suggested.

Case study 2

Angela was referred to the caseload team by one of the mainstream team midwives following her booking appointment early in pregnancy where it was reported that Angela had disclosed that she suffered from depression and had a history of self-harming and alcohol abuse. She stated that she had been under the care of the community mental health team (CMHT) but had refused to engage with them. She had also declined support from the drug liaison midwife – she said she hadn't wanted to be labelled as having an alcohol problem and was no longer drinking anyway. However, Angela had agreed to referral to the caseload midwives to provide her with some additional support.

When I met Angela for the first time, we met at her partner's flat where she was living at the time. Angela was very defensive and did not make eye contact. She did talk a little about her past though, and described how she had suffered from depression for several years – she was then 19 years of age. She had been on antidepressants and under the care of the CMHT since attempting to hang herself the previous year. However, she had taken herself off her medication and failed to engage with CMHT as she felt that it did not help her.

Angela's partner, Ian, was present throughout the visit and explained how he had a history of drug abuse and was currently being supported by the drugs team on a methadone programme.

The flat was in a very poor condition and would not have been suitable to having a baby live there. Angela and Ian stated that they had no motivation to clean the place up as they were moving to a larger flat nearby in the near future.

We discussed Angela's alcohol consumption and Angela admitted that she had been binge drinking prior to the pregnancy, but was not drinking at all since the pregnancy had been confirmed.

Angela expressed concern about whether there was a need for Social Services to be involved. It was explained that the services are there to provide help and support when it is needed and we openly discussed changes that could be made to the home and lifestyle to try to prevent the need for Social Services to be involved. Both Angela and Ian were very positive that they could make these changes, and were insistent that they wanted to turn their lives around and give their baby the best possible start in life.

And true to their word, over the coming months they moved into the new flat, and they took great pride in showing me each room that they decorated in turn. They prepared well for the baby, buying something each week, until they received the Sure Start maternity grant, which they used to buy the larger things for the baby, including a pram and cot.

I built up a good relationship with both Angela and Ian, and Angela regularly rang for information or advice. They kept all the appointments we made, and attended the required hospital appointments. Angela took great care of herself and showed a particular interest in eating healthily and getting regular exercise. She felt better with regard to her depression, but was aware that pregnancy and the postnatal period were a very vulnerable time for her, and she promised to ask for help if she needed it. Ian admitted to struggling with the methadone programme, but remained very determined.

By 32 weeks of pregnancy, it was evident that this young couple had made every effort to turn their lives around, and it was not considered necessary at that time, by myself or the health visitor, who I had also involved antenatally for additional support, to involve Social Services.

The pregnancy went to full term, and Angela gave birth, normally with no interventions or complications, to a baby boy weighing a healthy 7 lb 11 oz.

Angela and Ian had been very anxious about their lack of experience with regard to parenting skills, but both coped extremely well.

Five weeks following the birth they were continuing to cope well, enjoying being parents, and the flat remained clean and tidy. Their son was healthy and thriving and the family were discharged to the care of the health visitor.

Good practice point: bilingual maternity support worker

My role and responsibilities are to enhance antenatal and postnatal health, social care and parenting support for vulnerable women. I provide a support service based on the needs of the local community and also act as a resource for women with little or limited English.

By working closely with families I aim to improve outcomes for all children. I provide a service that will educate and support parents, helping them to address health needs and directing them to services that will provide support and a social network to prevent isolation. Good-quality care can make a substantial contribution to improving the immediate health and well-being of women and babies.

I work closely with local midwives to provide care to targeted families who have been identified as having a specific need for my support. I attend antenatal clinics to provide translation for women with little or no English and I also provide this service for midwives' antenatal and postnatal home visits. Sometimes, women are identified as having extra support needs, either by the midwife or myself at the antenatal clinic. This could be for a variety of reasons, but typically includes newly arrived women of South Asian heritage. During these home visits, I can make women aware of local community and social networks, for example, parent and toddler groups, antenatal groups, aquanatal sessions. These provide not only information but also social contact, lessening isolation and setting up a support network for after the birth of the baby. Encouraging women to engage with services is a key part of my role.

Whatever the circumstances, each woman and her family need to be approached and supported individually, with services tailored to their own situation. All maternity care providers should make every effort to be aware of all services that may be useful to their clients and be prepared to signpost these effectively.

To be 'with women' is the rhetoric of midwifery. Now we should be thinking of getting alongside her, to be with her and to support her as she moves into society's most important role, that of parent and teacher to the next generation.

(Hunt 2004, p. 7)

Key implications for midwifery practice

- What are the vulnerable groups in your area that are in need of additional support/service provision?
- What specialist midwifery services are in place in your area (drug liaison, teenage pregnancy etc.) and what is the scope for further development of these services?
- Consider how partnership working with other agencies may enhance maternity services in your area?
- Visit local children's centres and explore opportunities to provide more maternity services from these community venues.

- Involve local women and families in service development to ensure that the services being delivered meet the needs of local service users.
- Consider how recommendations from key reports and documents can be implemented in you area of work.
- Has the Common Assessment Framework been introduced by your local authority?

Notes

1 www.mind.org.uk/index.htm
2 http://www.languageline.com/

References

Babb P, Martin J, Heizewindt P (eds) (2004) *Focus on Social Inequalities*. London: Office for National Statistics.

Beake S, McCourt C, Bick D (2005) Women's views of hospital and community-based postnatal care: the good, the bad and the indifferent. *Evidence Based Midwifery* 3 (2): 80–86.

Beck C (2004) Birth trauma is in the eye of the beholder. *Nursing Research* 53: 1; Cited by Dearman S, Gutteridge K, Waheed W (2007) Maternal mental health: working in partnership. In: Edwards G, Byrom S (eds). *Essential Midwifery Practice: Public Health*. Oxford: Blackwell Publishing.

Beech B, Robinson J (1985) Nightmares following childbirth. *British Journal of Psychiatry* 147: 586.

Bick D (2008) Best evidence for maternal health? Midwives – RCM Magazine October / November.

Bick DE, MacArthur (1995) The extent, severity and effect of health problems after childbirth. *British Journal of Midwifery* 3 (1): 27–31.

Bostock Y (2003) *Searching for the Solution: Women, Smoking and Inequalities in Europe*. London: NHS Health Development Agency.

Bull J, Mulvihull C, Quigley R (2003) Prevention of low birth weight: Assessing the effectiveness of smoking cessation and nutritional interventions. *Evidence Briefing Summary*. Health Development Agency; Cited by Stringer E (2007) Health and inequality: what can midwives do? In: Edwards G, Byrom S (eds). *Essential Midwifery Practice: Public Health*. Oxford: Blackwell Publishing.

Byrom S, Downe S (2007) Narratives from the Blackburn West caseholding team: setting up. *British Journal of Midwifery* 15 (4): 225–227.

Cabinet Office (2006) *Reaching Out: An Action Plan on Social Exclusion*. London: HMSO. Available at: www.cabinetoffice.gov.uk/social_exclusion_task_force/publications/reaching_out.aspx (accessed 03/01/2009).

CEMACH (2004) *Confidential Enquiry into Maternal and Child Health 2000–2002*. London: CEMACH.

CEMACH (2008) *Perinatal Mortality 2006: England, Wales and Northern Ireland.* London: Confidential Enquiry into Maternal and Child Health.

Cox J, Murray D, Chapman G (1993) A controlled study of the onset prevalence and duration of postnatal depression. *British Journal of Psychiatry* 163: 27–41.

Darzi A (2008) *High Quality Care for All. NHS Next Stage Review Final Report.* London: The Stationary Office.

Dearman S, Gutteridge K, Waheed W (2007) Maternal mental health: working in partnership. In: Edwards G, Byrom S (eds). *Essential Midwifery Practice: Public Health.* Oxford: Blackwell Publishing.

Department for Children Schools and Families (2008a) *Health-Led Parenting Support.* Every Child Matters Update. Available at: http://www.everychildmatters.gov.uk/parents/healthledsupport/ (accessed 30/12/2008).

Department for Children Schools and Families (2008b) *Sure Start Children's Centres* Available at: http://www.surestart.gov.uk/surestartservices/settings/ surestartchildrenscentres/ (accessed 30/12/2008).

Department of Health (1998) *Independent Enquiry into Inequalities in Health.* London: HMSO.

Department of Health (2000) *Domestic Violence: A Resource Manual for Health Professionals.* London: The Stationery Office.

Department of Health (2003) *Tackling Health Inequalities: A Programme for Action.* London: The Stationery Office.

Department of Health (2005) *Responding to Domestic Abuse. A Handbook for Health Professionals.* London: The Stationery Office. www.dh.gov.uk/publications.

Department of Health (2006) *Responding to Domestic Abuse. A Handbook for Health Professionals.* London: Department of Health.

Department of Health (2007) *Maternity Matters: Choice, Access and Continuity of Care in a Safe Service.* London: HMSO.

Department of Health/Department for Education and Skills (2004) *National Service Framework for Children, Young People and Maternity Services: Maternity Services.*

Department of Health/Department for Education and Skills (2007) *Teenage Parents Next Steps: Guidance for Local Authorities and Primary Care Trusts.* London: HMSO.

Drife J, Lewis G (eds) (1998) *Why Mothers Die: Report on Confidential Enquiries into Maternal Deaths in the United Kingdom 1994–1996.* London: HMSO.

Fleming A (2008) *Blackburn with Darwen Midwifery Group Practice Quarterly Report*, July 2008 (unpublished).

Gateway Family Services (2008) Available at: http://www.gatewayfs.org/ pregnancy.html (accessed 01/03/2009).

Gaudion A, Allotey P (2008) *Maternity Care for Refugees and Asylum Seekers in Hillingdon. A Needs Assessment*: Centre for Public Health Research, Brunel University (internal report).

Hamlyn B, Brooker S, Oleinikova K, Wands S (2002) *Infant Feeding Survey 2000.* London: The Stationary Office.

Hepburn M (2005) Social problems in pregnancy. *Anaesthesia and Intensive Care Medicine* 6 (4): 125–126.

Hollings V, Jackson C, McCann C (2007) Teenage pregnancy: everyone's business. In: Edwards G, Byrom S (eds). *Essential Midwifery Practice: Public Health*. Oxford: Blackwell Publishing.

Huber U, Sandall J (2006) Continuity of carer, trust and breastfeeding. *MIDIRS Midwifery Digest* 16 (4): 445–449.

Hunt S (2004) All I want is a bit of respect. *Poverty, Pregnancy and the Healthcare Professional Books for Midwives*. London: Elsevier Science.

Kendell RE, Chalmers KC, Platz C (1987); Epidemiology of puerperal psychoses. *British Journal of Psychiatry* 150: 662–673.

Lavender T, Downe S, Finnlayson K, Walsh D (2007) *Access to Antenatal Care: A Systematic Review*. Available at: http://www.cemach.org.uk/Publications/CEMACH-Publications/Maternal-and-Perinatal-Health.aspx.

Leeds Asylum Seekers Network (2008) Available at: http://www.lassn.org.uk/befriending.htm (accessed 01/03/2009).

Lewis G (ed.) The Confidential Enquiry into Maternal and Child Health (CEMACH) (2007) *Saving Mothers' Lives: Reviewing Maternal Deaths to Make Motherhood Safer – 2003–2005. The Seventh Report on Confidential Enquiries into Maternal Deaths in the United Kingdom*. London: CEMACH.

McIver L (2007) Substance misuse: what is the problem? In: Edwards G, Byrom S (eds). *Essential Midwifery Practice: Public Health*. Oxford: Blackwell Publishing.

McLeish J (2002) *Mothers in Exile: Maternity Experiences of Asylum Seekers in England*. London: Maternity Alliance.

McLeish J (2005) Maternity experiences of asylum seekers in England. *British Journal of Midwifery* 13 (12): 782–785.

National Institute for Health and Clinical Excellence (2005) *Post-traumatic Stress Disorder (PTSD): The Management of PTSD in Adults and Children in Primary and Secondary Care*. Clinical Guideline 26.

National Institute for Health and Clinical Excellence (2006) *Routine Postnatal Care of Women and their Babies*. Clinical Guideline 37.

National Institute for Health and Clinical Excellence (2007) *Antenatal and Postnatal Mental Health Clinical: Management and Service Guidance*. Clinical Guideline 45.

Oates M (1996) Psychiatric Services for women following childbirth. *International Review of Psychiatry* 8: 87–98.

O'Hara MW, Swain AM (1996) Rates and risk of postpartum depression – a meta-analysis. *International Review of Psychiatry* 8: 37–54.

Oxford English Dictionary (2008). Available at: http://dictionary.oed.com (accessed 10/12/2008).

Prentice S (2007) Substance misuse in pregnancy. *Obstetrics, Gynaecology and Reproductive Medicine* 17 (9): 272–277.

Price S (2007) Domestic abuse in pregnancy: a public health issue. In: Edwards G, Byrom S (eds). *Essential Midwifery Practice: Public Health*. Oxford: Blackwell Publishing.

Richardson K (2001) *Smoking, Low Income and Health Inequalities: thematic Discussion Document Report for Action on Smoking and Health and The Health development Agency*; Cited by Stringer E (2007) Health and inequality: what can midwives do? In: Edwards G, Byrom S (eds). *Essential Midwifery Practice: Public Health*. Oxford: Blackwell Publishing.

Robertson E, Jones I, Haque S, Holder R, Craddock N (2005) Risk of puerperal and non-puerperal (postpartum) psychosis. *Short Report Br J Psychiatry* 186: 258–259.

Rowe R, Jayaweera H, Henderson J, Garcia J, Macfarlane A (2003) *Access to Care for Low Income Childbearing Women*. NPEU and Maternity Alliance.

Royal College of Midwives (1999) *Domestic Abuse in Pregnancy*. Position Paper 19. London: RCM.

Ryding E, Wijma K, Wijma B (1998) Predisposing psychological factors for post-traumatic stress reactions after emergency caesarean section. *Acta Obstetricia et Gynecologica Scandinavica* 77: 351–352; Cited by Dearman S, Gutteridge K, Waheed W (2007) Maternal mental health: working in partnership. In: Edwards G, Byrom S (eds). *Essential Midwifery Practice: Public Health*. Oxford: Blackwell Publishing.

Slater L, Byrom S (2006) Antenatal care in children's centres: making it happen. *RCM Midwives* 9 (11): 446–447.

Sutton C, Utting D, Farrington D (2004) ibid. Factors listed relate to risk of committing crime and anti-social behaviour. In Cabinet Office (2006) *Reaching Out: An Action Plan on Social Exclusion*. HMSO.

Swann C, Bowe K, McCormick G, Kosmin M (2003). *Teenage Pregnancy and Parenthood: A Review of Reviews, Evidence Briefing*. Sure Start, London: Health Development Agency.

White C (2007) New Generation of equality in perinatal care. *Health Service Journal*, November 2007.

Wieck A, Kumar R, Hirst AD, Marks MN, Campbell IC, Checkley SA (1991) Increased sensitivity of dopamine receptors and recurrence of affective psychosis after childbirth. *British Journal of Psychiatry* 303: 603–616.

Chapter 9
Working with Partners: Forming the Future

Selina Nylander and Christine Shea

> Health care is provided in partnership with patients, their carers
> and relatives, respecting their diverse needs, preferences and choices
> and in partnership with other organisations (especially social-care
> organisations) whose services impact on patient well-being.
>
> (Department of Health 2004)

Introduction

Health, social and voluntary care services in the United Kingdom
are increasingly being encouraged to work together across traditional
agency boundaries in an attempt to make the best use of resources
and to enable services to be responsive to the needs and views of the
communities they serve.

The maternity episode care is a period in which the distinction
between 'health' and 'social care' is frequently blurred, as a large
proportion of women who are pregnant, and who give birth in the
United Kingdom, progress through a natural physiological process,
which should not normally result in physical or mental ill health.

During the postnatal episode, women may receive care from a variety
of different professionals and healthcare workers. Women and their
families may also seek information and support from third parties
including the voluntary sector such as Home-Start (http://www.home-
start.org.uk) or holistic practitioners such as homeopaths. Each woman's
network of support will be unique to her and may involve different
individuals and professions providing support in parallel.

Maximising potential for health and social gain by working within
and across the professional boundaries has placed maternity care in

the forefront of the personalisation and partnership policy agendas. Chapter 5 provides a detailed description of how women and their families themselves become partners of the maternity care system both during and after their childbirth experience.

The importance and benefits of partnership working in maternity care, for both service users and providers of care, are discussed in this chapter. The work of midwives in partnership with other health professionals, voluntary sector organisations and women themselves in the immediate post-partum period and beyond is reviewed and debated. Old and new customs and research evidence are explored, in an attempt to identify and optimise the opportunities to provide appropriate and potentially bespoke support to the family unit during the postnatal period.

Maternity Matters (Department of Health 2007) gives relevance to this:

> High quality maternity care is not just about good professional care that ensures a healthy and safe pregnancy. It also involves access to a wide range of varied services that should work in partnership to help equip mothers and fathers with the skills they require to become confident and caring parents.

What is partnership working?

Partnership working is a term that is frequently used yet rarely defined. Within the National Health Service in the United Kingdom, the phrase is often used to describe a mechanism whereby service delivery is provided by two or more disciplines who work collaboratively to deliver optimal care for an individual. The Home Office (1992) defined partnership working as 'organisations with differing goals and traditions, linking to work together'. Other terms such as 'joint working' and 'collaborative care' are also used. For midwives, working in partnership within the organisation will mean working with the team involved in the care of the childbearing woman and her baby, such as obstetricians and paediatricians. In addition, midwives may also work in partnership with other statutory organisations, the independent sector and voluntary and third sectors during the maternity care episode.

In February (2008) The King's Fund published a document '*Safe Births: Everybody's business*', which reported on an independent inquiry into safety in maternity services. Whilst the inquiry focused on the intra-partum period, it emphasises the vital role of teamwork and collaboration in ensuring the safety of mothers and babies: 'Effective teamwork can increase patient safety; [while] poor teamwork can jeopardise safety.'

Several solutions to resolve difficulties in teamwork are suggested in The King's Fund report. These include ensuring clarity about team objectives and roles and that effective leadership is in place and clear and agreed procedures for communication are established.

Sometimes, by default but increasingly by design, different professions work in partnership successfully. However, the Audit Commission (2005) warns that this way of working does not always deliver value for money, and can sometimes cause confusion and hence weaken accountability, when insufficient attention is paid to questions of leadership, decision-making, scrutiny and risk management. Dickinson and Glasby (2008) also found that there is little clarity around both the definition of 'partnership' and the expected improvement in outcomes that should be seen after implementation of a successful partnership. These omissions undermine the success of the partnership and, as a result, the quality of care delivered.

As Cook *et al.* (2007) found in their work on the building of capacity in Health and Social Care Partnerships 'partnerships are a means to an end and not an end in themselves ... all stakeholder groups consulted agreed that the primary purpose of partnership working should be to deliver better outcomes to service users.'

Ultimately provision of a personalised maternity and postnatal service requires a formalisation of partnerships between agencies since 'the services that (go) furthest towards meeting quality-of-life outcomes for service users (are) those that work in partnership with a broader range of agencies, including housing, employment, and voluntary and private sector providers' (Petch *et al.* 2007).

Characteristics of partnership working

Partnership working generally occurs at two levels. There is a strategic level at which decision-making and joint planning occurs usually at the agency/organisational level. The second level is the implementation or service delivery. This is where the practical work between organisations occurs to provide integrated care. At this level, the partnership work may be formal as well as, quite often, informal when relationships have been built up between individuals within the different organisations. These relationships may be used to further improve patient care when shortcomings in formal partnerships become obstacles as opposed to enablers.

There is an expanding number of potential partners for midwives to collaborate with, thereby maximising potential for positive influence on women and families. These include the following:

Women using the service
Family members, for example, fathers and grandparents
Other members of the maternity team, for example, consultant
   obstetricians/paediatricians/anaesthetists

Health visitors and general practitioners (GPs)

The NHS and Social Services (including joint planning, commissioning and finance)

Voluntary agencies, for example, National Childbirth Trust (NCT), MIND, Association for improvements in maternity services (AIMS), Home-Start

Children's centres and Children's services

Private sector or third sector organisations, for example, doulas, independent midwives

Cross-sectoral and local government teams

Commissioning in partnership

Health care in the United Kingdom is increasingly planned and delivered as a 'joint' process. With more focus on 'upstream' thinking and preventative health care, the wider determinants of health are seen as important in planning for good health, rather than treating pathology as it arises. Services are 'commissioned' by Primary Care Trusts (PCTs), in response to local need.

The DoH White Paper – *Our Health, Our Care, Our Say: A New Direction for Community Services* (Department of Health 2006) – emphasised the need for the following:

- Greater integration of health and social care services outside hospitals with greater joint working through new commissioning partnerships between local authorities and reformed PCTs
- More control for individuals over their local health services to satisfy local need
- More involvement of patients in local commissioning decisions
- A shift in services towards prevention, for both ill health and admissions, and greater support for self-care

The most recent Department of Health driver for commissioners to establish 'World Class Commissioning' provides a clear vision that PCTs will need to work in demonstrable partnership to drive improvements across the highest priority services and meet the most challenging needs (Department of Health 2007).

Why work in partnership?

The fragmentation of service delivery, combined with changes in the structure of society, has led to women and babies becoming increasingly isolated from sources of support and succor at a time when they are fragile and vulnerable. Consequences for women when services are not coherently provided can result in postnatal morbidity and depression. The Confidential Enquiries into Maternal Deaths (CEMACH 2004, 2007) cite the failure of services to communicate with each other as a factor in some maternal suicides as GPs and psychiatric services often failed to provide information regarding previous histories of psychiatric disorders to maternity services. Had there been better communication, it is suggested that some of these deaths could have been prevented.

In the 2008 Cabinet office report, *Think Family: Improving the Life Chances of Families at Risk*, which was part of a Social Exclusion Task Force cross-Whitehall review on families at risk, it was advised that a 'system that "thinks family" has no "wrong door"; contact with any one service gives access to a wider system of support. Individual needs are looked at in the context of the whole family, so clients are seen not just as individuals but as parents or other family members. Services build on the strengths of families, increasing their resilience and aspirations. Support is tailored to meet need so that families with the most complex needs receive the most intensive support'.

Working in partnership in the immediate postnatal period

The majority of birth in the United Kingdom takes place in hospital, and the current service provision is resulting in early discharge home. The provision of coordinated care post discharge may mitigate/reduce a variety of negative health and welfare consequences for baby and mother. An example of this is the rapid decline in breastfeeding following the transfer of women home from hospital.

An early 'quick win' could be the improvement of both breastfeeding initiation and duration through improved coordination of hospital and post-discharge care.

A clinical review of breastfeeding by Hoddinott *et al.* (2008) stated that 'the biggest decline in breastfeeding occurs during the first four days after birth, when 12% of women in the UK stop, with 22% stopping by two weeks and 37% by six weeks'. Further work undertaken by the NCT found that 'nearly half of . . . . women [surveyed] said they did not receive as much support as they needed regarding breastfeeding [and] . . . . as a result of this, more than 50% of women stopped breastfeeding sooner than they would have liked (National Childbirth Trust 2006). Without improving the coordination and provision of support to these women a move towards earlier hospital discharge will continue to negatively affect this critical period during which breastfeeding success is established.

In a 2003 report *Evidence-Based Briefing on the Effectiveness of Public Health Interventions* to promote the initiation of breastfeeding National Institute for Clinical Excellence (NICE) (NICE 2003) found that peer support programmes as stand-alone interventions have been shown to be effective in both the antenatal and postnatal periods for women who expressed a wish to breastfeed, including those on low incomes. Chapters 5 and 7 provide examples of breastfeeding peer support programmes.

Working in partnership with families

A 'whole families approach' stresses the importance of looking at the family as a unit and of focusing on positive interdependency and supportive relationships (Cabinet Office Social Exclusion Task Force 2007). Better support of fathers and their active inclusion in their babies' birth and the postnatal health and welfare of mother and baby is a relatively new area of investigation and discussion. The contribution of the father and therefore the provision of support to facilitate the father's ability to support his partner and the baby is now viewed as a critical factor in improving babies' welfare – both short and long term. In a report by the Fatherhood Institute (2008), *The Dad Deficit: The Missing Piece of the Maternity Jigsaw*, evidence is presented to document the benefits to the child and parents of fathers' active and positive involvement from birth. More information is available on their website www.fatherhoodinstitute.org/. Providing knowledge in a suitable environment for the father could improve breastfeeding and consequently long-term health outcomes for both babies and mothers as this quote from the Treasury suggests:

> The UK Government believes much more can be done to release the potential improvements in outcomes for children through better engagement between fathers and services for children and families. This requires a culture change – from maternity services to early years, and from health visitors to schools – changing the way that they work to ensure that services reach and support fathers as well as mothers.
>
> (Department of Children, Schools and Families 2007)

Transfer of care: from midwife to health visitor

The National Service Framework for Children, Young People and Maternity Services (Department of Health 2004) states that women need to be provided with a postnatal care service that responds to their individual, physical, psychological, emotional and social needs and that this should be achieved through a multidisciplinary team-based approach. Whether giving birth at home or in hospital, once parents are on their own with their new baby at home, the first few days/weeks can be a huge adjustment, and for some it can be quite stressful. Antenatal preparation can be very important to prepare women and families for this period and to put in place plans to create an environment that will support the new mother, baby and father. As the trend to reduce the number of postnatal visits that women receive from midwives continues, the coordination and management of the transfer of care from midwife to health visitor becomes increasingly important.

In a study on transition to parenthood (Deave *et al.* 2008), the importance of continuity of care, both from the midwife and health visitor was stressed frequently by women, often because this was not achieved. Most significantly women in the study thought that the role of the midwife in the postnatal and post-hospital discharge period should be extended beyond 2 weeks to maintain the trust and consequently their own growing confidence as mothers that had started antenatally.

New initiatives have been trialed and recently implemented in the United Kingdom to strengthen and build on the historic links between Midwives and health visitors. The NICE guidelines on postnatal care (Department of Health 2007) are clear, noting that 'a coordinating healthcare professional should be identified for each woman. Based on the changing needs of the woman and baby, this professional is likely to change over time'.

This coincides with the introduction of the role of the 'lead professional', to head a multidisciplinary team in a Children's Trust, usually within a children's centre setting to support children and families with additional needs. The national framework for local change programmes, *Every Child Matters: Change for Children* (Department for Education and Skills 2004), aims to build services around the needs of children with an agenda for integrated front-line services, including the role of the lead professional. Lead professionals will support those children, young people and families who have additional needs that require input from more than one practitioner.

Most families with multiple problems are likely to have had considerable experience of mainstream services, such as the child's school or the family's GP, as well as contact with specialist services. However, their engagement with services may often have been chaotic and it requires a level of coordination beyond the capacity of the individual front-line worker or indeed that of the clients themselves (Cabinet Office Social Exclusion Task Force 2007).

The lead professional will deliver the following three core functions as part of their work:

- Act as a single point of contact for the child or family
- Coordinate the delivery of the actions agreed
- Reduce overlap and inconsistency in the services received

The importance of this partnership approach to the delivery of health care is emphasised in the Child Health Promotion Programme (CHPP) (Department of Health 2008) in which midwives and health visitors are required to work even more closely together. The CHPP is an early intervention and prevention public health programme that lies at the heart of the government's universal service for children and families.

Desired outcomes from the successful implementation of the CHPP are to encourage strong parent/child attachment and positive parenting, resulting in better social and emotional well-being among children and to increase rates of initiation and continuation of breastfeeding. Significantly, pregnancy and the first years of life are now being recognised as one of the most important stages in the life cycle, when the foundations of future health and well-being are laid down and a time when parents are particularly receptive to learning and making changes. Increasing levels of evidence suggest that the outcomes for both children and adults are strongly influenced by the factors that operate during pregnancy and the first years of life. Ensuring that children and adults are well supported through these years is a demanding task and clearly requires access and support to multiple services. Coordination and partnership is the only way to successfully meet this range of needs.

Children can be a big motivator for parents to change risk-taking behaviours. For example, a study of heroin-using mothers in Australia revealed that having a child was a key trigger for them to seek support and treatment to stop using drugs (Richter & Bammer 2000). Similarly, dealing with adult's needs enables them as parents to support and build resilience in their children as well as to reduce the risk that their children will go on to experience similar negative outcomes (Cabinet Office Social Exclusion Task Force 2007).

Children's centres are a way of delivering community-based services and are visible and accessible to families who might be less inclined to access traditional services. In addition, providing care through Children's centres means women and their families are able to access a range of other services and professionals whom they may otherwise have been unable to access.

The emphasis of the CHPP is recognition of the importance of pregnancy and the first 3 years of life in terms of later public health outcomes, in particular emotional health. Novel interventions are suggested with the integration of evidence provided within guidance for postnatal care from NICE (2007). The emphasis is on providing parenting support for the initial transition to parenthood and strategies to encourage strong couple relationships and father involvement. The CHPP focuses on outcomes, which are the same as those identified within the Public Service Agreement (PSA) priorities such as increasing breastfeeding rates, improving emotional health and reducing obesity.

While the CHPP sets out the expected standard for the child health promotion service, it does not dictate how the services are to be provided.

Working in partnership with communities

The debate in relation to this is fully explored in Chapter 5.

There are many examples on midwives working successfully in partnership with diverse ethnic groups to improve health and well-being, an example of this is the Liverpool LINK clinic (Box 9.1).

Box 9.1 Liverpool Link Clinic

The clinic was established to meet the needs of women who for cultural or religious reasons are unable to see a male doctor or who do not have English as their first language and would benefit from the support of bilingual health link workers (Akeju 2006). The clinic was developed in partnership and with input from focus groups of women from the diverse range of ethnicities it would support.

The aims of the service are to

- offer continuity of antenatal care within a non-judgemental framework from a small group of midwives;
- increase attendance at antenatal clinic and reduction of problems associated with women from ethnic minority women, for example, women who have undergone female genital mutilation (FGM) and have low levels of calcium and vitamin D;
- offer parent education in liaison with health link workers and interpreters;
- endeavour to have a holistic approach to health for the benefit of mothers and babies.

Akeju (2006) found that informal feedback from women and midwives suggested that the services offered give vulnerable women continuity of care in the antenatal period and enable early detection and resolution of problems and she felt that the service acted as a flagship of partnership.

Different approaches to nurturing new mothers

In many cultures the isolation and lack of support experienced by some mothers in the United Kingdom is simply eliminated through communal approaches to postnatal care in which there is a tradition of caring for new mothers for 40 days, with ceremonies to welcome the woman and her newborn back into the community. Many health workers and anthropologists believe that women from traditional cultural backgrounds with large kin groups exhibit fewer symptoms of postnatal depression (Stern & Kruckman 1983) as a result of this care and attention. Pillsbury (1978) found that the physical and emotional stresses following childbirth are well identified and managed by rituals in an indigenous community, so that the experience and likelihood of depression is minimised.

An interesting social support mechanism is the henna traditions within Islam, Sephardic Judaism, Hinduism and Coptic Christianity, which may play a significant part in the management of post-partum depression in India, North Africa and the Middle East (Cartwright Jones 2002). Henna's association with beautification and protection from evil are comforting to pregnant women. Younger girls are often included in these rituals which reinforce the roles and responsibilities inherent in motherhood, support a woman's journey to motherhood by reducing fear and provide a predictable source of emotional and physical support from family members and friends before, during and after birth. The accepted and well-established partnerships and pattern of responsibilities inherent in such cultures further facilitate the mother's well-being. The basic requirement that a woman be still for several hours during and after application of henna insures that a mother will rest and allow others to take care of her. Henna rituals performed in the late stages of pregnancy establish a woman's 'social safety net' within her community. Participation confirms those who will help her through birth and with reintegration into the community after childbirth. During the weeks after ornate henna patterns are applied, a woman is allowed to refrain from household tasks that would spoil the beauty of the stains. Following the ritual postnatal henna ceremony, this increases the likelihood that she will rest properly to regain her strength after giving birth while relying on others to provide her with support and manage her household.

Working in partnership with general practitioners: practice-based commissioning and the role of the GP in postnatal care

Practice-based commissioning (PBC) is a government policy initiative that devolves responsibility for commissioning services from PCTs to local GP practices. Under PBC, practices are given a commissioning budget, which they will have the responsibility for using in order to provide services. This will involve the following:

- Identifying patient needs
- Designing effective and appropriate health service responses to those needs
- Allocating resources against competing service priorities

The key objectives of PBC are to

- improve clinical engagement;
- provide better quality, more convenient services for patients;
- bring about more efficient use of resources.

General practice is increasingly aware of the influence of social and cultural factors on health and several new types of treatment are becoming available from GPs to treat conditions such as postnatal depression. One of these is social prescribing, a mechanism for linking patients in primary care with non-medical service support in the community. Friedli and Watson (2004) state that social prescribing has benefits in three key areas:

1. Improving mental health outcomes
2. Improving community well-being
3. Reducing social exclusion

This model of treatment could help to reduce inequalities and improve well-being for postnatal women.

One example of this is the NHS social prescribing community initiative (set up by Rossendale Enterprise Anchor Ltd (REAL) in partnership with NHS East Lancashire), which includes exercise or arts on prescription, referral to community-based self-help groups, befriending schemes and volunteering opportunities. It also includes support with benefits, debt, legal advice and parenting problems. Another new therapy, available to GPs, sets a new green agenda for mental health. Mind (The National Association for Mental Health in the United Kingdom) has called for ecotherapy to be recognised as a clinically valid treatment for mental health problems and a core component of an adequate public health strategy for mental health. Ecotherapy has been found to directly benefit mental health (lowering stress and boosting self-esteem), improve physical health (lowering blood pressure and helping to tackle obesity), provide a source of meaning and purpose, help to develop skills and form social connections (Pretty *et al.* 2005, 2006, 2007). This could be specifically useful for women who do not want to take antidepressants (including those who are breastfeeding).

Working in partnership with the third sector

The third sector describes a range of institutions, which occupy the space between the state and the private sector. These include local community and voluntary groups, large and small registered charities, foundations, trusts and the growing number of social enterprises and co-operatives.

Third sector organisations share common characteristics in that they are

- non-governmental;
- 'value-driven' that is, primarily motivated by the desire to further social, environmental or cultural objectives rather than to make a profit per se;
- principally reinvest surpluses to further their social, environmental or cultural objectives.

The government and health sector are increasingly recognising the role of third sector organisations – building social capital, engaging communities and providing a campaigning voice advocating for change and informing the development of government policy.

The social enterprise approach is being recognised by the government as 'a way forward for community and voluntary sector (CVS) organisations'. A social enterprise is a business with primarily social objectives whose surpluses are principally reinvested for that purpose in the business or in the community, rather than being driven by the need to maximise profit for shareholders and owners.

Many social enterprises look beyond traditional public service delivery mechanisms developing services that address the needs – whether of an individual or the community – in a much more holistic and joined up way.

The NHS in the United Kingdom has invested in third sector approaches, particularly social enterprise, which they believe, help to put people in control of their health care, and offer patients and users a greater choice from a wider selection of convenient, innovative and responsive services.

The Third Sector Strategy and Action Plan (DFES 2007) found that the third sector historically develops services that are flexible and innovative and engage users, especially those who may find it difficult to articulate their needs or who may be harder to reach through mainstream provision.

Parents can be reluctant to engage with mainstream health and social care services for many reasons, including the following:

- Disillusionment in services unavailable, inappropriate or unacceptable

- Fear and lack of trust in (authority)
- Humiliation (not wanting to admit they need help)

Voluntary sector organisations may act as a buffer or advocate between families and health professionals. Third sector organisations are often particularly well placed when it comes to working with families at risk because of their detailed local knowledge of the issues faced by excluded families and because of their approachability in the eyes of family members (Cabinet Office Social Exclusion Task Force 2007).

A survey by Henricson (2001) of family services found that the voluntary sector provides 49% of family support services. One organisation that works with parents in the United Kingdom is Home-Start. This is a confidential home-visiting scheme offering emotional support, friendship and practical help to families with a child younger than 5 years. Volunteers visit families in their homes for as long as they are needed.

In one of the charities' reports 'Learning from Families' they concluded that 'It could be argued that all families lie along a continuum of disengagement/engagement, and they can move in either direction in response to services and policies'. In this study they found that in spite of notable exceptions among health visitors, GPs, consultants and other service personnel, in general parents felt that 'People in authority knock your self-esteem and are not good at explaining or taking parents' worries seriously'. Yet, one parent described their experience of Home-Start:

> I can trust Home-Start. The volunteers and staff are always there and you can talk to them. It is like being with your mates. We have a good laugh. It never feels official.
>
> (Homestart 2005)

Another very well-established third sector organisation that works with parents is the NCT. The NCT has been working with pregnant women and families since 1956.

The NCT is the UK's leading charity on pregnancy, birth and early parenthood and they support parents from bump to baby. Each year they support thousands of parents through a life-changing experience, offering expert information and trusted practical and emotional support through their network of 300 local branches, help lines, antenatal and early days classes, breastfeeding, counselling and peer support schemes. Recognised by parents for more than 50 years, the NCT campaigns continuously strive for improvements to maternity care and better services for all new parents. They work to make becoming a parent a more positive experience and help parents to be the parent they want to be.

The NCT base their information and support on research evidence and the views of parents. As a result, they are viewed by many as independent experts in matters relating to pregnancy, birth and early parenthood and are an influential and trusted advisor to UK governments, royal colleges, private sector bodies and other charities. Much of the charity's work is in conjunction with other partners, whether they be the NHS, Children's Centres or other agencies. NCT teachers are currently delivering services in such diverse locations as Styal Prison where they run antenatal classes; Wai Yin Chinese Women's Society in Manchester where they have run antenatal classes with the aid of an interpreter and will soon be running an early day's course and the Countess of Chester hospital where, like Birmingham Women's Hospital and other hospitals across the United Kingdom, the NCT has won a contract to deliver all of the antenatal education.

The charity's mission statement states that the charity supports all parents and it is showing its commitment to reaching out to all parts of the community, particularly through its Reaching Out projects. Since 2005, the NCT has been working with a small charity called Sowing Seeds, funded through the Parenting Fund, on supporting men and fathers around Manchester, and building a network for parenting practitioners in the Northwest to share good practice. In the West Midlands, a Department of Health grant is funding the NCT to support women living in deprived and rural areas locally who are from black and minority ethnic (BME) groups, teenage parents and women suffering domestic violence. The charity also funds more than 60 outreach projects each year for families on low income, those with disabilities, teenagers and lone parents.

For further information go to www.nct.org.uk or call NCT Enquiries on 0300 330 0770.

Another example of an organisation that fills the gaps that statutory services can leave for women and families is the AIMS. This charity was established in 1960 and acts as a campaigning organisation that provides information on parents' rights, a confidential helpline and publishes a quarterly journal. AIMS has campaigned in the past for the following:

- Fathers to be admitted to the labour wards
- Ending routine procedures such as pubic shaving and enemas
- Women's right of access to their case notes and records
- Major reductions in the routine episiotomy

When women mistrust health and social care agencies, organisations such as AIMS provide a safety net for access to support. They frequently anticipate and campaign for change; for example, AIMS acknowledged and published that mothers often hid the truth when health visitors screened them for postnatal depression, before research and other expert information was available.

Other agencies and charities can also offer support for women and their families. An example of this is in Liverpool in the United Kingdom, where close collaborative working among Liverpool Women's NHS Foundation Trust, Liverpool PCT and the National Society for the Prevention of Cruelty to Children (NSPCC) has resulted in the creation of two midwifery specialist posts that are supporting women and families who are affected by substance misuse and/or domestic violence.

The Birth Trauma Association (BTA) was established in 2004 to support women or their partners suffering from postnatal post-traumatic stress disorder (PTSD) or birth trauma. A British study by Warwick University and Northampton General Hospital, published in *Psychology, Health & Medicine* in 2003, quotes a PTSD rate in women after childbirth of 2 to 5%. It is estimated that, in the United Kingdom alone, this may result in 10,000 women developing PTSD in a year. Also, as many as 200,000 more women may feel traumatised by childbirth and develop some of the symptoms of PTSD.

> PTSD is also far more complicated than postnatal depression because it is a direct result of a woman's trauma, yet, she may feel bound to be grateful to the very people who violated her and caused that trauma.
>
> (Kitzinger 2003)

Whilst it is difficult to hear that some women feel psychologically harmed by their labour experience, it is important that their stories are heard and acknowledged, as this can help women to move on with their lives and also provides a deeper understanding of the care practices and procedures that can lead to PTSD and help prevent this occurring to other birthing women in the future. For further information go to www.birthtraumaassociation.org.uk/

In order to guarantee continuity of care, sometimes after a previous traumatic birth, some women choose to opt out of some aspects of NHS care, accessing information or support through the internet, hiring an independent midwife or a doula.

Independent midwives are fully qualified midwives who, in order to practice the midwife's role to its fullest extent, have chosen to work outside the NHS in a self-employed capacity, although they support its aims and ideals. The midwife's role encompasses the care of women during pregnancy, birth and afterwards working one to one in partnership with the woman providing the midwifery component of their maternity care. Currently, women pay directly for this service but independent midwives in the United Kingdom (formally the Independent Midwives Association (IMA)) with the government's support are becoming a social enterprise in order to contract the services of their members into PCTs so that this option of care would be available to any pregnant woman. This is indeed what the IMA have been campaigning for over many years. They proposed a partnership model of care (NHS Community Midwifery Model (NHSCMM)) based on how they have traditionally worked to be available to women through the NHS.

A doula provides continuous, emotional and practical support for pregnant women, new mothers and their families during the time around childbirth. She is usually a mother herself and may also have undertaken a period of preparation to work as a doula, although this is not mandatory. Doulas may specialise in supporting women through pregnancy, labour and birth (birth doulas), or in the time shortly after birth (postnatal doulas) or they may work in both areas. Doulas do not perform clinical or medical tasks; they provide information/signposting to support informed choice and emotional and practical support to women and their families. Established in 2001, Doula UK Ltd is a non-profit organisation run voluntarily by doulas for doulas. The network aims to set a 'gold standard' amongst the doula community through provision of the Doula UK Recognition Process. This is an initial period of independent assessment and mentorship to be undertaken by all new doulas, usually further to completion of a Doula UK Recognised Course. The organisation works to promote the role of the doula, encourage communications between doulas, and advance their understanding of birth and the postnatal period. Members work within the guidance of the Doula UK Code of Practice and Philosophy, and all have access to Doula UK's Hardship Fund established in 2002 to support disadvantaged women. The network is overseen by Doula UK's Doula Council, which includes a number of eminent midwives and birth activists. In the case of unsupported women or women who are in prison, some doula services are offered on a voluntary basis. See www.doula.org.uk for more information.

More than 15 studies have been carried out around the world, demonstrating the many benefits of hiring a doula, including a Cochrane review (Hodnett *et al.* 2003).

A doula's presence during birth has been found to

- shorten first-time labour by an average of 2 hours;
- decrease the chance of caesarean section by 50%;
- decrease the need for pain medication;
- help fathers participate with confidence;
- increase success in breastfeeding (Klaus *et al.* 1993).

Additional findings attributed to the support of the postnatal doula show improved parent–baby bonding and decreased incidence of postnatal depression.

A number of volunteer doula programmes have been set up to work within the NHS and with disadvantaged communities, including Birth Companions, a charity providing a doula service for pregnant women in Holloway prison. See www.birthcompanions.org.uk/ for more information.

Homerton Birth Companions (known as Birth Buddies) was set up to support Black African and Afro-Caribbean women during pregnancy and labour. International research suggests that such support can be beneficial for birth outcomes. An evaluation of the programme in reducing infant mortality (Department of Health 2008) found that Birth Buddies provided valuable reassurance for women while they were in labour, helping them to relax and calm them and enabling women to cope with their labour.

Partnership working for change in maternity services

Partnership can also be an effective model to drive change in maternity services. NHS organisations have a statutory obligation to consult the public about proposed changes and every PCT should have its own Maternity Services Liaison Committee (MSLC), which is an independent advisory body comprised of representative clinicians from all specialties involved in maternity care, together with relevant commissioners, managers, public health and social care input and at least one-third user members, bringing together their different perspectives in partnership to plan, monitor and improve local maternity services. These committees can be an excellent example of successful partnership work in practice, or sometimes the opposite, exhibiting the weaknesses and barriers common to partnership work.

The One Mother One Midwife (OMOM) campaign is an example of where mothers and midwives together drive forward the case for change.

OMOM is a group of mothers, fathers and midwives who have joined together to campaign for change in maternity services by government implementation of the IMA proposed 'NHS Community Midwifery Model' (NHSCMM.) This will provide one-to-one continuity of care and choice for women of all socio-economic classes within the United Kingdom.

The model of NHS community midwifery care would enable any woman to have the option to choose one-to-one care throughout her pregnancy, labour and the postnatal period from a midwife of her choice. This model would sit alongside the current midwifery service and it would be up to each woman which model she would choose. Similar systems currently work in New Zealand (http://www.maternity.org.nz/choices.shtml) and parts of Canada, based in the community, ensuring equity of access for all women and are recognised as being at the forefront of international maternity provision. Since this model was introduced, over half of all women from New Zealand choose a midwife practising independently as their lead maternity professional for their pregnancy, birth and the postnatal period.

By providing equitable access to maternity services, which is particularly important for vulnerable groups, for all women; Chapter 8 provides accounts and examples of working to address this subject.

Conclusion

In this chapter, we have defined partnership working, described its importance and proposed the potential for improving maternity care. We have also discussed the benefits of a combined approach to campaigning for change in maternity services. Some of the consequences of a failure to work in partnership and the processes and requirements for successful partnership working have been discussed.

The postnatal period is a complex period of time. The newborn has to adjust to life outside the womb, establish its first attachments, learn to eat, sleep and develop. Women progress through childbirth as a rite of passage to motherhood and all that it entails. Men become fathers dealing with the differing demands of the twenty-first century, to provide and nurture a new family unit, which is created within the wider community. It is only through working in partnership with others that midwives will meet the differing needs of those in their care. Midwives have a magic moment of opportunity to influence the future of our species, and what is more important than that?

> Human conversation is the most ancient and easiest way to cultivate the conditions for change – personal change, community and organizational change, planetary change. If we can sit together and talk about what is important to us, we begin to come alive. For as long as we've been around as humans, as wandering bands of nomads or cave dwellers, we have sat together and shared experiences. We've painted images on rock walls, recounted dreams and vision, told stories of the day, and generally felt comforted to be in the world together. When the world became fearsome, we came together. When the world called us to explore its edges, we journeyed together. Whatever we did, we did it together.
>
> (Margaret Wheatley 2002)

Key implications for midwifery practice

- Find out how many practice-based commissioning groups are in your area and what areas they are concentrating on. Can you influence the topics?
- What local organisations also offer support to pregnant women and their families. Does your maternity service work in partnership with these?
- Check that your maternity services are welcoming to fathers, particularly young fathers.
- Find out if midwives have a voice in influencing the commissioning cycle. What is commissioned locally? Is this appropriate for women's needs?
- Engage with your local third sector agency to see how you work together to provide additional support for women and their families.
- What are the breastfeeding initiation rates in your hospital? What groups are available locally to support breastfeeding women? What are the rates at transfer to the community and at 6 weeks after birth?
- Are there any practice-based commissioning projects in your area? What involvement do midwives have in the initiatives? Could you refer women in your care for social support?
- Find out how the Child Health Promotion Programme is being implemented in your area. Where are the Children's centres in your area of practice? How are local midwives engaging in the children's centre agenda?
- Are there doulas working in your local area? Consider signposting women who may benefit from their extra support.
- Have you attended the MSLC in your area? Could you encourage women in your care to get involved in your area's MSLC?

References

Akeju D (2006) The link clinic: promoting innovative practice through partnership. *British Journal of Midwifery* 14 (7): 412–414.

Audit Commission (2005) *Governing Partnerships: Bridging the Accountability Gap*. London: Audit Commission.

Cabinet Office Social Exclusion Task Force (2007) *Reaching Out: Think Family*.

Cartwright Jones C (2002) *Traditional Postpartum Rituals of India, North Africa, and the Middle East: Seclusion, Henna, & 40 Day Homecare*. Kent, Ohio: Medical Anthropology, Kent State University.

CEMACH (2004) *Why Mothers Die 2000–2002*. London: CEMACH.

CEMACH (2007) *Saving Mothers' Lives 2003–2005*. London: CEMACH.

Cook A, Petch A, Glendinning C, Glasby J (2007) Building capacity in health and social care partnerships: key messages from a multi-stakeholder network. *Journal of Integrated Care* 15 (4).

Deave T, Johnson D, Ingram J (2008) Transition to parenthood: the needs of parents in pregnancy and early parenthood. *BMC Pregnancy and Childbirth* 8: 30, doi:10.1186/1471-2393-8-30.

Department for Children, Schools and Families (2007) *Aiming High for Children: Supporting Families*. London: Treasury.

Department of Health (2004) *National Service Framework for Children, Young People and Maternity Services Standard 11: Maternity Services*. London: Department of Health.

Department of Health (2006) *Our Health, Our Care, Our Say: A New Direction for Community Services*. London: Department of Health.

Department of Health (2007) *World Commissioning: Vision*. London: Department of Health.

Department of Health (2008) *Child Health Promotion Programme (CHPP): Pregnancy and the First Five Years*. London: Department of Health.

Department for Education and Skills (2004) *Every Child Matters: Change for Children*. London: Department for Education and Skills.

Dickinson H, Glasby J (2008) Not throwing out the partnership agenda with the personalisation bathwater. *Journal of Integrated Care* 16 (4).

The Fatherhood Institute (2008) *The Dad Deficit: The Missing Piece of the Maternity Jigsaw*. www.fatherhoodinstitute.org/index.php?id=2&cID=734 (accessed 11/2008).

Friedli L, Watson S (2004) *Social Prescribing for Mental Health*. Durham: Northern Centre for Mental Health.

Henricson C, Katz I, Sandisin M, Tunstill J (2001) *National Mapping of Family Services in England and Wales*. London: National Family and Parenting Institute.

Hoddinott P, Tappin D, Wright C (2008) Breast feeding. *British Medical Journal* 336: 881–887.

Hodnett ED, Gates S, Hofmeyr GJ, Sakala C (2003) Continuous support for women during childbirth (Cochrane review). *The Cochrane Library* 3.

Home Office (1992) *Partnership Working in Dealing with Offenders in the Community*. London: Home Office.

Homestart (2005) *Learning from Families, Policies and Practices to Combat Social Exclusion in Families with Young Children in Europe, Sheila Shipman*. http://www.home-start.org.uk/about/Final_EW_Report_Summary_smaller.pdf (accessed 30/11/08).

The King's Fund (2008) *Safe Births: Everybody's Business King's Fund London*. www.kingsfund.org.uk/publications/kings_fund_publications/safe_births.html.

Klaus MH, Kennell JH, Klaus PH (1993) *Mothering the Mother: How a Doula Can Help You Have a Shorter Easier and Healthier Birth*. Reading, MA Perseus Books, 168 pp.

Kitzinger S (2003) Kate Hilpern *The Guardian*, Wednesday 28 May 2003. http://www.guardian.co.uk/lifeandstyle/2003/may/28/familyandrelationships.health

National Childbirth Trust (2006) *Midwives Top Chart for Breastfeeding Information*. www.nct.org.uk/press-office/press-releases/view/13 (accessed 11/2008).

National Institute for Clinical Excellence (2003) *The Effectiveness of Public Health Interventions to Promote the Initiation of Breastfeeding*. London: NICE.

National Institute for Clinical Excellence (2007) *Postnatal Care: Routine Postnatal Care of Women and their Babies*. London: NICE.

Petch A, Miller E, Cook A, *et al.* (2007) *Users and Carers Define Effective Partnerships in Health and Social Care*. Department of Health. http://www.masc.bham.ac.uk/Reports/UCDEP.pdf.

Pretty J, Hine R, Peacock J (2006) Green exercise: the benefits of activities in green places. *The Biologist* 53 (3): 143–148.

Pretty J, Peacock J, Hine R, *et al.* (2007) Green exercise in the UK countryside: effects on health and psychological well- being, and implications for policy and planning. *Journal of Environmental Planning and Management* 50: 211–231

Pretty J, Peacock J, Sellens M, *et al.* (2005) The mental and physical health outcomes of green exercise. *International Journal of Environmental Health Research* 15 (5): 319–337.

Pillsbury BLK (1978) "Doing the Month": confinement and convalescence of Chinese women after childbirth. *Social Science in Medicine* 12: 11–12.

Richter KP, Bammer G (2000) A hierarchy of strategies heroin-using mothers employ to reduce harm to their children. *Journal of Substance Abuse Treatment* 19 (4): 403–413.

Robinson J (2007) Thoughts of hurting the baby. *AIMS Journal* 19 (3).

Stern G, Kruckman L (1983) Multi-disciplinary perspectives on postpartum depression: an anthropological critique. *Social Science in Medicine* 17: 1027–1041.

Wheatley M (2002) *Turning to One Another: Simple Conversations to Restore Hope to the Future*. San Francisco Berrett-Koehler Publishers.

Chapter 10
Nurture and Nature: The Healthy Newborn

Annie Dixon

Introduction

Many changes have occurred over the last decade in terms of how families and the newborn are supported and cared for. Successive policy documents such as *The Children's Act* (UK Government 2004), *Every Child Matters* (DfES 2004), the *National Service Framework* (DoH 2004), *Working Together to Safeguard Children* (DfES 2006) and *The Children's Plan* (DfES 2007a) have culminated in the introduction of the Child Health Promotion Programme (DoH 2008a). This programme integrates many of the complexities and the dynamic, multilayered facets involved in raising children. However, the plan retains the distinctiveness of each aspect that facilitates healthcare workers[1] (HCWs) to provide optimal support to parents during pregnancy through to the fifth year of their child's life.

New parents rarely understand how having a child can change life and all parents seek reassurance that their infant is healthy and developing as expected. Parents sometimes require support to become competent and confident in carrying out the practical skills of parenting, such as feeding. Therefore, key aspects of a midwife's postnatal practice include supporting development of practical skills, providing anticipatory guidance and promoting and facilitating positive parenting.

This chapter discusses some of the important features involved in caring for the newborn, with a special emphasis on nurture, nutrition and screening. Although the focus is on the support that can be provided by midwives and other HCWs, there should be recognition and encouragement of the use of multi-agency partners who are able to support and nurture the parenting process.

Nurturing and responses

Transition to parenthood

Mothers and fathers are likely to adapt to parenthood in different ways and at different times (Dulude *et al.* 2000). For women, transition can start to occur as soon as the pregnancy is confirmed whereas for men the process may only begin to become real when they see the ultrasound scan of their unborn child (Draper 2002; Cooper 2005). Transition to parenthood can be stressful (Mercer *et al.* 1988; Newman & Newman 1988; Maloni *et al.* 2001) as both internal identity (self) and external relationships (with others) are modified to embrace the new arrival (Hackel & Ruble 1992; Kreppner 1988; Partridge 1988).

Healthcare practitioners can, and do, influence the ease of this transition (Meleis 1997). For families who have to remain in hospital, either for maternal or infant care, consideration should be given to ensuring that the family feels involved and supported in caring effectively for their newborn. It may be difficult for parents to be completely at ease within the hospital environment as their perceived level of control may be reduced. One strategy that can be used to alleviate this is for HCWs to explore where the parents are on the novice-to-expert parenting continuum. Discussing a parent's previous experience and knowledge with them will enable information to be provided in the most effective way. Everything may be new for first-time parents whereas for experienced parents the infant will be new but the basic principles of caring for a baby will already be known. However, a parent's experience or competence should never be assumed. New parents may have gained experience of childcare through other family members or work and yet practice changes over time, and hence the current approach to childcare may be very different for them.

Parent–infant relationships

Parent–infant attachment (Bowlby 1969; Ainsworth *et al.* 1978) is another crucial facet of a healthy family. The choice of the word 'parent' is deliberate as the term mother–infant attachment leaves out at least one-third of the intact family unit – the partner. Traditionally, mothers have been seen as the primary caregivers (Ferri & Smith 1996) and thus the term mother–infant attachment was coined. One outcome from this was the marginalisation of fathers. Taylor and Daniel (2000) suggested that such marginalisation leads to the mother being seen as the focus of attention and that the potential of the father as either an asset or a risk goes unnoticed.

The development of a father's role from simply being a provider and disciplinarian has occurred steadily over the last few decades due to societal, cultural and economic changes. The influence that fathers have on every domain of their child's development should not be underestimated (Coleman *et al.* 2004). For example, newborns will often turn their heads towards their father's voice in preference to the voice of a stranger (Brazelton 1992), and where a father is the main caregiver they become the primary attachment figure (Geiger 1996). Given this, it is imperative that HCWs not only acknowledge and celebrate the contribution fathers make to family life but also actively seek to integrate them into their infants' care (DfES 2007b; DoH 2008a). Box 10.1 provides some tips and strategies for including fathers, and for more detailed support a visit to the fatherhood institute website would be beneficial (Fisher 2007).

Box 10.1 Tips and strategies for including fathers

Remember to be father friendly by
- having inclusive policies and practices;
- welcoming fathers and speaking to them directly rather than directing everything to the mother;
- exploring how the father perceives his role and looking at ways of integrating that into the care being given;
- actively engaging the father by including him in decision-making.

Childbirth can be extremely tiring and new mothers should be assessed to gauge the amount of support, help, reassurance and rest they need. Historically, infants were placed in nurseries so that the mothers could rest. Current practice recommends that infants stay with their mothers to avoid the potential issues arising through separation. The option of early discharge for the healthy mother–infant dyad helps to preserve the natural family unit although it provides little time for education or support prior to discharge home. Historically, the extended family and good social networking within the community would have provided the support required. Current lifestyles, however, leave some new mothers coping alone once home, apart from the visits from the midwife and/or health visitor. Extended families are not always close by and community cohesion is variable (Muntaner *et al.* 2000). Therefore, some new mothers in the community may require additional support and reassurance to replace this. Women need to be alerted to these issues antenatally so that they can ensure adequate support is available when discharged.

Healthy family dynamics

Whether in the hospital or community setting, families will interact with a number of HCWs and other agencies. For HCWs to effectively support nurturing behaviours within and between the different relationships of a family unit there are several aspects of family that must first be discussed.

Family structures

Firstly, the meaning of 'family' may mean different things to different people. Academics may define 'family' differently depending on their theoretical perspective. Governments tend to focus on the structure–function aspect of family, which encompasses those individuals involved in raising their children (DfES 2007b). This is necessary for legislative and supportive mechanisms to be effective; however, it does not encompass the vast array of individual differences in perception. Some individuals may choose to define their family based on their situation, psychosocial-biological needs and their interaction with others. Families within society today may consist of the traditional mother- and father-led families, single-parent families (either mother- or father-led), same sex parent families and blended families (includes step parents). All of these different family structures require the same degree of respect and support from HCWs.

Cultural aspects of care

When providing care and support for families, HCWs must be mindful of the issues that can arise from differing cultural backgrounds as these can influence outcomes. Cultural issues are highly complex and multilayered; for example, individual cultural beliefs are interlaced within family culture, family beliefs are interlaced within the community culture and/or workplace culture, and so on. Personal beliefs stem from all aspects of a person's life, such as, their primary language, strengths, social networks, parenting style, religious preference and life experiences. Other cultural groupings, such as family, community, workplace and profession will have their own set of beliefs to which individuals become encultured. Given that parenting is a complex activity, comprising behaviours that affect the overall development of the infant in a variety of ways including their emotional, physical, social, and neuro-development, it is crucial that HCWs respect a family's culture and work alongside a family's beliefs rather than against them. The objective is not to change the worldview of the family but to provide the best evidence-based care possible within their worldview (Seibert *et al.* 2002). This can sometimes be difficult as different cultural 'norms' can appear strange and incomprehensible because of a lack of understanding of where the belief comes from. However, most cultures hold some common values despite perceiving some behaviour in very different ways. Consequently, HCWs should be willing to develop their understanding of the differing cultural beliefs, values and norms that they encounter to provide effective, culturally sensitive care and support. The first step in achieving this is for HCWs to be aware of their personal values, attitudes and beliefs through reflecting both personally and professionally (Leonard & Plotnikoff 2000). Secondly, HCWs need to be aware of how different cultures perceive health, well-being and illness as this will impact on a person's recovery and compliance. Thirdly, an understanding and non-judgemental acceptance of the family's culture and how care can be managed to best meet the family's needs is essential. Only when all of these aspects are integrated can the care provided be holistic and culturally competent (Bhui *et al.* 2007).

Positive parenting

Once the HCW has established how a particular family functions and their underlying cultural perspective, then parental concerns can be addressed effectively to provide support and promote positive parenting. As stated earlier, parenting skills are not innate and parents can be empowered through support and education to provide a positive and healthy family environment for the optimum development of their children. Many parents have concerns regarding not only the practical skills involved in parenting but also the less tangible skills of positive parenting, and there are a variety of resources available to enable HCWs to support parents effectively (FPI 2008; NSPCC 2008). Initially, one of the most important things a HCW can do is to promote and enable healthy family dynamics (Skinner *et al.* 2000; Tammentie *et al.* 2004; Sanders & Woolley 2005). This can be achieved in a number of ways. A simple strategy such as providing positive encouragement and support, through the mindful use of communication Burgoon *et al.* (2000), to strengthen the parents' belief in themselves and their ability to parent effectively can be used. More complex strategies such as motivational interviewing (MI) provides supportive talk to aid a person's understanding of the thought processes so that emotional reactions can be identified and then challenged to facilitate the introduction of alternative behaviours (Bundy 2004). The three pivotal aspects of MI are to adopt the main principles of the person-centred approach (Rogers 1953) in a directive way by using the Stages of Change model (Prochaska & DiClemente 1982) in conjunction with the guiding principles for successful MI (Rollnick *et al.* 2007). A systematic review of MI found it to be effective, even in sessions of less than 20 minutes duration (Rubak *et al.* 2005) and the level of effectiveness was increased if repeat encounters took place. This evidence would suggest that HCWs would benefit from training in MI to enable them to provide optimal support to parents.

Responding to parental concerns

Even when parents have received all the reassurance they need, other aspects of having a new baby can impact family functioning.

Sleep deprivation

Babies wake up in the night for feeds and for some families this broken sleep can continue for a long period of time. Sleep deprivation can have a devastating effect on a person's ability to cope, their sense of self-esteem and their mood (Bonnet & Arand 2003). New parents, and especially mothers, require reassurance that how they are feeling is normal. In situations where sleep loss is affecting their physical or mental ability to cope, referral for additional support services would be appropriate. The government has pledged that every family will be able to access support through a children's centre by 2010 (DoH 2007a) and this framework would be advantageous as in many areas multiple services would be grouped within the centre and for the most disadvantaged families outreach workers would provide the support required.

Co-sleeping

The practice of co-sleeping is used by parents either intentionally or unintentionally for a variety of reasons (Hooker *et al.* 2001; Ball 2003). Parents may believe that their infant will sleep better if they are co-sleeping and there is a strong relationship between co-sleeping and mothers who breastfeed (Blair & Ball 2004). Historically, co-sleeping was discouraged as it was thought to increase the incidence of Sudden Infant Death Syndrome (SIDS) but more recent research has suggested the risk is greater for parents who smoke (Carpenter *et al.* 2004).

Co-sleeping with infants less than 11 weeks old carries a greater risk of SIDS even when factors such as smoking are taken into account (Adler *et al*. 2006) and therefore HCWs must provide evidence-based information for families that is congruent with their local policy (RCM 2004).

Positive touch

There are measures parents can instigate that will have a beneficial impact on family life. Parents can be given information and guidance on the best ways of providing age-appropriate stimulation for their baby to help development in a variety of domains such as social interaction, motor, and brain development (Bidmead & Mackinder 2004). Educating parents to look for and understand their baby's behavioural cues will empower parents to provide stimulation or support appropriate to the baby's state (Bidmead & Andrews 2004). When parents can assess their baby's behavioural state they will be able to introduce positive touch in the most effective way and this will also help both mothers and fathers to develop a deeper bond with their baby (Bidmead & Farnes 2004; Lorenz *et al*. 2005).

Nutrition

Breastfeeding

Evidence confirms that breastfeeding is beneficial to the infant and mother with regards to both short- and long-term health (Kramer & Kakuma 2002; Hoddinott *et al*. 2008). The vast majority of women are able to breastfeed successfully if they are well-informed and realistic about

a) how to establish breastfeeding;
b) wanting to breastfeed;
c) how long establishing breastfeeding will take;
d) getting support from their partner/family;
e) coping with sections of society that may not encourage breastfeeding.

Breastfeeding may be best but few women realise that patience will be needed to establish breastfeeding. There is growing evidence to suggest that early skin to skin care following birth facilitates breastfeeding as it enables the infant to become familiar with the smells and voices of their parents (Moore *et al*. 2007). The 2005 Infant Feeding Survey (Bolling *et al.* 2007) suggested that there had been an increase in the number of mothers initiating breastfeeding and yet the number of mothers still breastfeeding at 6 weeks was comparable to that found in the 2000 survey. The survey stated that mothers provided a variety of reasons for stopping breastfeeding in the first 2 weeks following birth and the most common reasons were as follows:

1. The baby was not sucking or the baby rejecting the breast
2. An insufficient milk supply
3. Suffering with painful breasts or nipples
4. That breastfeeding took too long or was too tiring

The number of women citing insufficient milk increased by 17% between weeks one and two within the survey data. Birth order also appeared to influence the success rate of breastfeeding. First-time mothers more commonly stated rejection of the breast as a reason whereas multi-parous women were more likely to give domestic reasons for stopping.

Another common concern of breastfeeding mothers is how much milk their baby is receiving. Women can be reassured that if their infant is producing wet nappies and is gaining weight then they will be getting the nutrients and fluid they need to grow and develop. It is important to educate mothers about how their baby will grow when breastfed. The World Health Organisation (WHO) has developed growth charts based on information from breast-fed babies to better reflect their growth patterns rather than the rapid weight gain of a bottle-fed infant (BBC 2007). These are currently being piloted in Scotland with a view to rolling them out nationally next year.

A knowledgeable breastfeeding mother is much easier to support as she will understand that her baby may want to feed more often because breast milk is more easily digested than formula milk. Therefore, it is crucial that HCWs enable parents to understand the process of breastfeeding a baby and that each local area has agreed policies and practices so that women are given the same information and support (McInnes & Chambers 2008). There may be instances when a HCW and parent will not agree and the HCW should respect the parental views whilst using every opportunity to educate and inform parents of evidence-based practice in terms of nutrition and feeding. It may be useful for peer and professional supporters to have some knowledge and understanding of the range of parenting approaches available to parents so that mindful information and support that may have more chance of influencing attitudes and behaviours can be suggested. For example, in certain approaches parents are encouraged not to feed their infants more often than every 3 hours. In a breast-fed infant this could result in hunger, lack of increased production of milk during growth spurts and the longer term failure of the infant to thrive. Hospitals and communities can work towards achieving Baby Friendly Status (BFI) to help increase breastfeeding rates, and further information on this can be found in Chapter 7.

Mothers need support, encouragement and reassurance to establish and maintain breastfeeding successfully. Timely information for sore nipples or ways to increase milk production will help mothers to continue exclusive breastfeeding for 6 months as recommended by the WHO (2002).

Tongue tie

One physiological problem that can affect breastfeeding success is ankyloglossia (tongue tie). This congenital anomaly is characterised by an abnormally short lingual frenulum. The result of this is that the tip of the tongue cannot protrude past the lower incisors. The severity ranges from mild to severe. In its mild form, the tongue is attached to the floor of the mouth by a thin mucous membrane whereas in the severe form the tongue is fused to the floor of the mouth. The majority of tongue ties do not need any treatment and some resolve over time. However, for mothers wishing to breastfeed, tongue tie can interfere with effective attachment, thus reducing the infant's ability to feed successfully. There are a number of non-surgical approaches that can be used to alleviate this issue including breastfeeding advice from a lactation consultant, massaging the frenulum and tongue exercises (AAP 2004; Watson Genna 2007), although their usefulness is questionable (Hogan *et al.* 2005). The main problem with these approaches is that if they do not work quickly then the ability of the infant to breastfeed successfully is compromised and may never recover sufficiently for exclusive feeding to continue. Where a tongue tie is impacting on attachment, surgical division soon after birth would ameliorate this problem with little risk to the infant. Some midwives are now being trained to perform this simple procedure, and guidance is provided by the National Institute of Clinical Excellence (NICE, 2005).

Artificial feeding

Despite both the physical and emotional benefits of breastfeeding, approximately a quarter of women choose to formula feed (Bolling *et al.* 2007). Those who choose this method of feeding should be afforded the same level of respect and support provided to breastfeeding women.

Formula feeds are usually based on cow's milk and the protein they contain is either whey or casein based. Non-cow's-milk formula, for example, soy-based formula, is not recommended for infants under 6 months of age unless there is a specific reason for it to be given. Casein-based formula, for example, follow-on milk, is not recommended for infants under 6 months as it is less easily digestible (Bolling *et al.* 2007).

Given that nearly a quarter of women choose to initiate feeding with formula milk and that by week 6 of life over three quarters of infants will have received some formula milk, (Bolling *et al.* 2007) it is imperative that HCWs offer education, reassurance and support to mothers on the sterilisation of equipment and making-up of feeds. As powdered milk is not a sterile product and the equipment used to make formula feeds is handled by mothers in domestic kitchens, formula milk can contain microorganisms that may pose a risk to the health of the infant. Therefore, strict guidelines should be followed when sterilising equipment and making up feeds. Parents should be given information and education on sterilisation and making up formula feeds to ensure the mother is competent and confident in preparing feeds prior to discharge. However, evidence would suggest that despite the information given, women often choose not to follow the guidelines provided. Nationally, less than a third of mothers followed all of the recommended guidance with older, more educated women complying with the guidance less often than younger more socially disadvantaged mothers (Bolling *et al.* 2007). This poses a challenge for HCWs as the common assumption may be opposed to reality. A good starting point would be to give all women the leaflet produced by the Department of Health on sterilising equipment and making up feeds (DoH 2008b) so that the relevant aspects can be discussed more fully with the family prior to discharge and again in the community if required. It should also be remembered that women may not always understand or read leaflets and so alternative methods such as demonstrations should be available for families to access.

Screening

Infant health is of paramount concern and the newborn undergoes a variety of procedures to ensure that optimum health is maintained. The Child Health Promotion Programme identifies the screening that a newborn will receive and the most beneficial timing for the tests (DoH 2008a).

What is screening?

Screening is a way of assessing if an individual, within a defined population, is at risk of a particular condition (NSC 2000). There are set criteria used to help decide which conditions would benefit the population by initiating a screening programme (NSC 2003), including looking at the condition, the test to be used, the treatment and the screening programme. Conditions suitable for a screening programme must be well defined and have a clear incidence within the given population. Additionally, for screening to be beneficial and cost-effective there should be a reduction in mortality or morbidity with associated improved health outcomes through treatment and/or information following the screening process. If screening suggests that an individual is at risk, then diagnostic investigations will be necessary to confirm or eliminate the condition. Screening programmes make a valuable contribution to public health but they can provide false positives (an erroneously positive result) and false negatives (an erroneously negative result). Parents need to be advised of this in a format that they can understand. False negatives are problematic as necessary treatment could be delayed. The Child Health Promotion Programme (DoH 2008a) stipulates that local areas should have agreed pathways with the information and systems in place to ensure that screening can be carried out in a timely, effective manner. This enables audits to measure how well standards are being met in order to ensure that an excellent service is offered to parents and their family.

Parental information on screening

Explaining newborn screening to parents involves more than providing information on the nature of a test. In order for parents to give informed consent, the details provided must include how the screening will be done, why it will be done and the meaning of the results obtained. The concept that tends to be most difficult for HCWs to explain is risk. Risk is about the probability or chance of something occurring, and HCWs have to appreciate the inherent uncertainty of this concept if they are to explain it in a way that will be valuable to parents. Risk is the *potential* for something to happen. Think of it in terms of risk management at work. A risk assessment of controlled drugs will look at how they are managed and highlight areas where there is the potential for an error to occur. Policies can then be devised to minimise the risk. This is the same idea as screening. A screening test takes information it knows to be true (research evidence suggesting incidences of conditions within given populations) and then looks at how likely it is that any one individual might have that condition. This may sound straightforward but other aspects of communication need to be factored in to ensure that risk has been understood appropriately by parents.

As explained earlier, each person has life experiences, values and fundamental beliefs that have developed from the society and cultures that they have been exposed to. All of these contribute towards an individual's personality and attitudes. These, in turn, impact on how information is provided, received and perceived. To check out your own perception, see Activity 10.1.

Activity 10.1: Perceptions of risk

1. Below are four statements. Two are written in percentage terms and two written as ratio data. Read all four and then choose which *one* you prefer.

   a) One in four people will experience mental illness during their lifetime.
   b) Twenty-five per cent of people will experience mental illness during their lifetime.
   c) Seventy-five per cent of people will not experience mental illness during their lifetime.
   d) Three in four people will not experience mental illness during their lifetime.

2. When you have chosen your preferred statement think about why you chose this one instead of any of the others. What was it that drew you to this particular choice?
3. What do the reasons for your choice tell you about how you view the world?
4. Does how you view the world influence how you present information to parents?
5. How do you think others may view the world?
6. Given that not everyone perceives things in the same way how might this influence how you present information on risk to parents in future?

A simple and well-used example is the half-filled glass. When presented with a half-filled glass, some people will see it as half-full and others as half-empty. Those in the half-full group are considered optimists, whereas those who perceive the glass to be half-empty are considered pessimists. Taking this one step further, optimists may think that a one-in-four chance of a potential problem might seem like really good odds as it means that three times out of four there is no problem. Similarly, if there is a one-in-two chance, an optimist may still believe that these are fairly good odds as half the time there is no problem. On the other hand, pessimists may see a one-in-four chance of a potential problem as worrisome and a one-in-two chance may be perceived as having a very good chance that there will be a problem. Therefore, it is important to gain a sense of not only *how* parents understand the information provided but also what *contextual framework* they are placing the information in.

The above example is fairly simplistic but the rarity of some conditions that are screened for add layers of complexity that need to be taken into account. For example, phenylketonuria (PKU) only affects 1 in 10 000 people. A parent presented with this figure alone might believe that the risk is so low as to not warrant the blood test to find out. However, PKU is a serious disease because if phenylalanine levels accumulate in the body the development of the brain will be affected, leading to learning difficulties. As it is entirely manageable through diet, the best practice would be to begin treatment as early as possible to prevent any problems. Newer tests enable laboratories to screen for less rare conditions such as sickle cell diseases (SCD) and cystic fibrosis (CF), both of which affect approximately 1 in every 2500 people. Within the United Kingdom, 1 in 20 people are CF carriers (Rushforth & Kini 2003), and 1 in 10 Afro-Caribbeans are sickle cell (SC) carriers (GenePool 2006). Neither of these conditions can be cured, but early intervention and knowledge that a person has them is beneficial to their long-term health.

It is important to remember that screening looks at risk; it does **not** provide a diagnosis of a condition.

Parental consent must be gained prior to carrying out screening procedures as it is vital that parents accurately understand the nature of the test. Activity 10.2 provides an opportunity to explore the concept of informed consent.

Activity 10.2: Informed consent

Write down or gather the information together that you would provide to parents if you were going to inform them about the blood spot test.

Does this information provide them with everything they need to know?

- Concept of risk
- Possibility of inaccurate result
- What is going to be tested for
- What each condition is and what can be done for it
- When they will hear the results
- Answer any questions they have
- What if they do not want all the tests
- Will they have to sign a consent form
- What will happen next

To ensure that parents have fully understood the information given to them, it is good practice to ask them to repeat the information given and their understanding of it. This way any misconceptions or gaps in knowledge can be corrected. HCWs should be aware of local and national policies as well as professional accountability in terms of gaining consent. Some areas have agreed that verbal consent is sufficient whereas other areas may require written consent for certain tests. Additionally, HCWs who rotate on a neonatal unit need to be aware that the consent process may be different from the postnatal wards.

Screening tests

Immediately following birth, the Apgar score may be assessed to provide information on the cardiorespiratory condition of the infant. However, many maternity units have abandoned its use in favour of more detailed resuscitation documentation as the usefulness of the Apgar score is controversial and extremely subjective (AAP & ACOG 2006). To date, nothing has been devised to replace this scoring system at birth. The midwife or doctor will assess the infant to ensure that no external gross abnormalities such as extra or missing digits, cleft lip and/or palate, and so on can be seen. All of this information provides a baseline for the infant, from which all subsequent measurements can be compared to evaluate their growth and development.

The first formal neonatal examination takes place between 4 and 72 hours of birth (Hall & Elliman 2006). This will be done by a HCW trained to carry out newborn examinations competently, with the relevant clinical experience, in the hospital or in the community (Townsend *et al.* 2004). Where a mother has taken early discharge, it is particularly important that fail-safe procedures are in place to ensure that the newborn examination is carried out in the community. This eight-step routine examination is thorough and detailed to screen for any conditions and examine for any abnormalities that require further investigation. National standards and competencies (NSC 2008a) have been produced to reduce variation in practice and ensure a quality service. Table 10.1 provides an overview of the eight steps and the components within each step.

The newborn examination provides an ideal opportunity for health promotion activity through anticipatory guidance (Bethell *et al.* 2001), to explore if any additional services or support may be needed due to other family illness or disease, and, last but not least, to provide information on other services and/or agencies that may be useful to the family (Hall & Elliman 2006).

Changing roles and blurring of boundaries has led to some midwives enhancing their skills by undertaking additional training in order to conduct newborn examinations. Research suggests that mothers are

Table 10.1 Eight steps to comprehensive newborn examination (CNE).

1. Awareness of national and local policies, guidelines, standards and competencies relevant to CNE
2. Provide information to parents and gain parental consent
   Provide written and verbal information on the following:
   - Process
   - Timing
   - Components of the examination
   - Limitations of screening
   - Risks
   - Outcomes
   - Further sources of information

3. History gathering
   - Maternal case notes – relevant prenatal and intra natal risk factors
   - Infant case notes
   - Family history
   - History taking

4. Physical examination

Head and ears	Fontanelles
	Head circumference facial features – symmetry
	Position of ears in relation to facial features
	Neck – swelling
Eyes	Red reflex
	Position
	Size
	Symmetry
Mouth	Tongue tie
	Soft and hard palate
	Teeth
	Vanula
Skin	Intact
	Birthmarks, dimples or rashes
	Colour
	Webbing
Respiratory system	Bilateral equal air entry
	Bilateral chest movement
	Size and shape of check and nipple position
	Breathing rhythm and rate and depth
Cardiovascular system	Auscultation of heart sounds
	Pulses – peripheral and femoral
	Evidence of oedema
	Hepatomegaly
Abdominal palpation	Observation of abdomen – shape, soft or tense on palpation
	Presence of organomegaly
	Presence of bowel sounds
	Palpable bladder
Spine	Intact
	Palpation
	Presence and level of sacral dimple – blind or open ended, assessment of depth
	Sacral tufts

(*continued*)

Table 10.1 (*continued*)

Extremities	Number of digits
	Position
	Colour
	Presence and degree of talipes – congenital or positional
Hips	Ortolani–Barbur manoeuvre
	Subcluxation/dislocation of hip/hips
	Assessment of limb length
	Symmetry of posterior and anterior limb creases
Genitalia	Sex determination
	Imperforate anus
	Descended/undescended testes
	Central urinary meatus
	Hypospadias or hydrocele
	Vaginal tags
Reflexes	General tone
	Neurological reflexes
	Neuro-behavioural assessment
	Sleep state
	Assessment of cry
5. General well-being assessment	
Nutrition	Type of milk – breast, formula
	Type of feeding – exclusive, complementary, scheduled, demand
	Method – breast, bottle, cup, tube
	Frequency
	Weight gain
Gastrointestinal tract	Urine output – amount, frequency, colour, smell
	Bowel motion – amount, frequency, colour, consistency

6. Anticipatory guidance /health promotion information
   - Vitamin K
   - Parent–infant attachment
   - Positive parenting strategies
   - Maternal and infant dietary requirements
   - Postnatal depression – signs/symptoms
   - Infant milestones
   - Signs for infant concern
   - Prevention of SIDS
   - Vaccinations/immunisations
   - Car seats
   - Smoking
   - BCG and Hep B vaccination – high-risk populations
   - Safety aspects
7. Parental feedback – discuss outcome of examination with parents and answer any questions they have
8. Documentation – contemporaneous. Offer appropriate, effective and timely referrals where necessary

Undertaken at <72 hours and <8 weeks by a trained, competent healthcare worker.
Compiled from National Standards and Competencies (NSC 2008a).

more satisfied when midwives perform the newborn examination as they are better at doing them (Wolke *et al.* 2002; Bloomfield *et al.* 2003). However, a study by Townsend *et al.* (2004) suggested that a significant number of midwives are not using this skill. One reason for this may be staffing constraints; yet, best practice and optimum care of infants would suggest that midwives, who are trained and proficient, should be undertaking this practice. Apart from meeting the needs of the changing agenda of maternity services, midwives can offer a more holistic approach to the care of the well neonate. Cost–benefit analysis may demonstrate a benefit to trusts whose midwives and neonatal nurses (rather than senior house officers) undertake newborn examinations and as such may help towards putting forth a case for more resources/midwives.

Many infants will experience physiological jaundice (hyperbilirubi-naemia) within the first week of life (Munro Cohen 2006). This occurs due to increased levels of unconjugated bilirubin circulating through the body due to the breakdown of haemoglobin from red blood cells, whose life cycle is shorter in the newborn than in the older child (Stevenson *et al.* 2001). This, coupled with the immaturity of the liver's ability to metabolise the unconjugated bilirubin into conjugated bilirubin, leads to infants displaying the classic yellow discolouration of the skin (Hansen 2007). However, it is important to be aware that if the onset of jaundice occurs within the first 24 hours of life or if jaundice is prolonged (pathological jaundice), the underlying cause should be investigated (Deshpande 2008). All infants with jaundice require observation to ensure that the unconjugated bilirubin does not exceed advisable levels as this may lead to bilirubin encephalopathy. Initially, a non-invasive method of testing bilirubin levels may be used such as the degree of jaundice visible to the naked eye. If warranted, a blood sample can be sent to the laboratory to provide an accurate picture of the clinical situation so that the appropriate management can be initiated, either conservative treatment, for example, phototherapy or more aggressive treatment, for example, exchange transfusion.

Between days 5 and 8 of life, the newborn blood spot screening is collected (preferably on day 5 of life). National screening for PKU and congenial hypothyrodism (CHT) has been routine for many years, although effective local implementation has been variable. This test has now expanded to include screening for SCD and CF. Most areas of England now test for medium-chain acyl-CoA dehydrogenase deficiency (MCADD) and this will be offered in all areas of England by 2009. It is important that health professionals are aware of what is tested for in their own locality, especially given that the government targets for reducing health inequalities (DoH 2008c). There are currently nine national standards for blood spot screening, as shown in Table 10.2 (NSC 2008b).

Table 10.2 Screening standard for blood spot test adapted from NSC 2008c.

Standard 1	Completeness of offer
Standard 2	Enhanced tracking abilities
Standard 3	Timely sample collection
Standard 4	Timely sample dispatch
Standard 5	Quality of blood sample
Standard 6	Timely receipt of a report/second blood spot sample
Standard 7	Timely processing of screen positive samples
Standard 8	Timely identification of babies for whom the Child Health Record Department has not received notification of specimen received in laboratory, screening test result or decline
Standard 9	Completeness of uptake

There is a vast array of information available on how to effectively collect the blood for this test and all relevant health professionals should avail themselves of this information (NSC 2008c). Poorly collected samples will need to be repeated. Delays of this nature put infants who are subsequently diagnosed with a condition, at risk of not receiving treatment within the expected time frame. Additionally, having to repeat sampling increases the stress for the parents and infant as well as increases the HCW's workload. Attention to detail can help minimise this.

Infant hearing has been tested since the 1960s, when health visitors would use the infant distraction test (reliant on the infant responding to sound). As this was partly dependant on infant behaviour as well as hearing, some infants needed unnecessary follow-up and others with hearing problems were undetected. Advances in technology have made it possible for screening for hearing to be undertaken at an earlier age and with increased sensitivity and specificity so that since 2006 all parents have had the infant hearing test recommended to them. This test is done before the infant is 4–5 weeks old using the automated otoacoustic emission (AOE) screening test where the echo that the cochlea emits after receiving a sound is noted. This service is offered in a majority of maternity units prior to the discharge of the mother and infant; alternatively, the test is available in the community. One or two infants in every 1000 have some hearing loss in one or both ears and the evidence would suggest that the earlier an intervention programme is introduced, the better the outcome for the infant in terms of language acquisition, speech, social and emotional development (DfES 2003). However, as no screening test is 100% reliable, parents should also be given a checklist that will enable them to assess if their baby is reacting appropriately to sounds at different stages of their development. They should be advised to seek professional help if they are concerned about their baby's hearing at any time. Sometimes an infant may have to have more than one hearing test and this may be due to something as simple as the baby being unsettled, a lot of background noise being present, or fluid or a temporary blockage in the ear after birth which usually resolves on its own over time. An alternative to the AOE test is the automated auditory brainstem response screening test (AABR). This test may take longer to perform than the AOE and can last up to 30 minutes.

The comprehensive physical examination of the infant is usually repeated between 6 and 8 weeks of age. This is to check that the infant is developing as expected and to ensure that no concerns remain undetected such as cardiac anomalies, a high soft palate cleft or congenital dislocation of the hip (Knowles *et al.* 2005). Age-appropriate health promotion information can also be provided to parents at this time.

Alongside these routine screening procedures, parents are also offered a variety of other relevant preventative interventions. All parents are offered the opportunity for their infants to be given Vitamin K, as one in 1000 infants are at potential risk of bleeding due to deficiency of Vitamin K. The newborn screening website suggests that Vitamin K should be given within 1 week of birth, and yet this would not prevent the early onset form from occurring. Ideally, vitamin K should be given soon after birth as recommended by NICE clinical guidelines (NICE 2006) and route and frequency of administration depend on the method of feeding. Breastfed babies require subsequent doses to address the perceived belief that breast milk contains low levels of vitamin K, whereas bottle-fed babies receive their continued requirements via formula milk. The route of administration also impacts upon the efficacy of vitamin K, with the intramuscular route being preferable due to the depot effect in the muscle of the oral route.

Infants whose mothers are carriers of hepatitis B or who have other family members living in the household with hepatitis B will be vaccinated within 2 days of birth and again at 1 month and 2 months of age. This will be followed by a booster dose and further tests at 1 year of age (DoH 2008d). Parents of infants who are at greater risk of contracting tuberculosis (TB) will be offered the opportunity of having their baby immunised for TB, especially if they will be travelling to a TB-active region such as India.

All infants will continue to be monitored and parents will continue to receive support and information through the child health programme until the child reaches 5 years of age.

Conclusion

The three main topics covered in this chapter are individually important to the healthy development of future generations. However, for optimal progress all three are interdependent.

Ongoing programmes of research and policy generation provide information on the best evidence-based practice. Locally agreed guidelines can facilitate consistency in the support and information provided to families. If HCWs are to utilise this effectively, continuing personal and professional development is crucial. In support of this, commissioners and providers can foster practice that is targeted towards the needs of individual families more effectively, thus moving towards a more efficient, sustainable and responsive service. Ongoing service evaluation will enable families and the health service to work together whilst celebrating diversity and social inclusion.

The hope is that this chapter has begun to demonstrate how HCWs can provide a holistic package of care for infants in partnership and collaboration with their parents and families.

Key implications for midwifery practice

- Healthcare workers must ensure that in caring for the family, all significant parties are included; mother, child and father/partner as all are integral to enabling healthy family dynamics and positive parenting.
- Parenting skills are not innate; mothers and fathers need education, support and reassurance to facilitate competence in practical skills such as feeding and psycho-social skills such as nurturing their infant within a healthy family dynamic.
- HCW have a duty to engage in mindful practice to ensure that they deliver culturally competent care.
- Early diagnosis of ankyloglossia (tongue tie) is crucial as it can affect the establishment of breastfeeding. Midwives trained to undertake frenulotomy whilst adhering to local guidelines can alleviate this difficulty.
- Screening is poorly understood and explained. Further training and ongoing discussion is necessary.
- Research suggests that mothers are more satisfied with midwives carrying out the newborn examination; yet, a proportion of midwives trained to carry out this procedure do not do so routinely.

Notes

1 Healthcare workers include midwives, doctors, health visitors, nursery nurses and so on.

References

Adler MR, Hyderi A, Hamilton A (2006) Clinical inquires: what are safe sleeping arrangements for infants? *The Journal of Family Practice* 55 (12): 1083–1084, 1087.

Ainsworth MDS, Blehar MC, Waters E, Walls S (1978) *Patterns of Attachment: A Psychological Study of the Strange Situation.* Hillsdale: Erlbaum.

American Academy of Pediatrics (2004) *Breastfeeding: Best for Baby and Mother.* Summer: AAP. Available at: http://aap.org/breastfeeding/8-27%20Newsletter.pdf (last accessed 10/10/2008).

American Academy of Pediatrics and American Committee of Obstetricians and Gynaecologists (2006) The Apgar score. *Pediatrics* 117 (4): 1444–1447.

Ball H L (2003) Breastfeeding, bed sharing and infant sleep. *Birth* 30 (3): 181–188.

Bethell C, Peck C, Schor E (2001) Assessing health system provision of well-child care: the promoting healthy development survey. *Pediatrics* 107 (5): 1084–1094.

Bhui K, Warfa N, Edonya P, McKenzie K, Bhugra D (2007) Cultural competence in mental health care: a review of model evaluations. *Health Services Research BioMed Central* 7: 15.

Bidmead C, Andrews L (2004) Enhancing early parent–infant interaction. Part one: observation strategies. *Community Practitioner* 7 (10): 387–389.

Bidmead C, Farnes J (2004) Enhancing early parent–infant interaction. Part two: positive touch. *Community Practitioner* 7 (11): 434–436.

Bidmead C, Mackinder L (2004) Enhancing early parent–infant interaction. Part three: early play. *Community Practitioner* 7 (12): 471–473.

Blair PS, Ball HL (2004) The prevalence and characteristics associated with parent-infant bed sharing in England. *Archives of Disease in Childhood* 89 (12): 1106–1110.

Bloomfield L, Rogers C, Townsend J, Wolke D, Quist-Therson E (2003) The quality of routine examinations of the newborn performed by midwives and SHO's; an evaluation using video recordings. *Journal of Medical Screening* 10 (4): 176–180.

Bolling K, Grant C, Hamlyn B, Thornton A (2007) *2005 Infant Feeding Survey.* London: The Information Centre.

Bonnet MH, Arand DL (2003) Clinical effects of sleep fragmentation versus sleep deprivation. *Sleep Medicine Reviews* 7 (4): 297–310.

Bowlby J (1969) *Attachment.* New York: Basic Books.

Brazelton TB (1992) *Touchpoints: Your Child's Emotional and Behavioural Development.* Reading: Addison-Wesley.

British Broadcasting Corporation (2007) *Baby Growth Chart Switch Closer.* BBC News Online 13th August, http://news.bbc.co.uk/1/hi/health/6943949.stm (last accessed 21/09/2008).

Bundy C (2004) Changing Behaviour: using motivational interviewing techniques. *Journal of The Royal Society of Medicine* 97 (Suppl. 44): 43–47.

Burgoon JK, Berger CR, Waldron VR (2000) Mindfulness and interpersonal communication. *Journal of Social Issues* 56 (1): 105–127.

Carpenter RG, Irgens LM, Blair PS *et al.* (2004) Sudden unexplained infant death in 20 regions of Europe: case control study. *Lancet* 363 (9404): 185–191.

Coleman WL, Garfield C, Committee on Psychosocial Aspects of Child and Family Health (2004) Fathers and pediatricians: enhancing men's roles in the care and development of their children. *Pediatrics* 113 (5): 1406–1411.

Cooper S (2005) A rite of involvement?: men's transition to fatherhood. *Durham Anthropology Journal* 13 (2): 1–24. Available at: http://www.dur.ac.uk/anthropology.journal/vol13/iss2/cooper/cooper.pdf (last accessed 27/07/2008).

Department for Education and Skills (2003) *Developing Early Intervention/Support Services for Deaf Children and their Families*. London: DfES.

Department for Education and Skills (2004) *Every Child Matters: Change for Children*. London: DfES.

Department for Education and Skills (2006) *Working Together to Safeguard Children: An Executive Summary*. London: TSO.

Department for Education and Skills (2007a) *The Children's Plan*. London: DfES.

Department for Education and Skills (2007b) *Every Parent Matters*. Nottingham: DfES.

Department of Health (2004) *National Service Framework for Children, Young People and Maternity Services: Executive Summary*. London: DoH.

Department of Health (2007a) *Delivering Health Services through Sure Start Children's Centres*. London: DoH.

Department of Health (2008a) *Child Health Promotion Programme*. London: DoH.

Department of Health (2008b) *Bottle Feeding*. London: DoH.

Department of Health (2008c) *Tackling Health Inequalities. Status Report on the Programme for Action*. London: DoH.

Department of Health (2008d) *Hep B vaccine NHS Immunisation Information*. London: DoH. Available at: http://www.immunisation.nhs.uk/Vaccines/Travel_*and*_other/Hepatitis_B/Hep_B_-_Vaccine (last accessed 19/09/08).

Deshpande PG (2008) *Breast Milk Jaundice*. eMedicine, http://www.emedicine.com/ped/TOPIC282.HTM (last accessed 17/10/2008).

Draper J (2002) 'It was a really good show': the ultrasound scan, fathers and the power of visual knowledge. *Sociology of Health and Illness* 24 (6): 771–795.

Dulude D, Wright J, Belanger C (2000) The effects of pregnancy complications on the parental adaptation process. *Journal of Reproductive and Infant Psychology* 18 (1): 5–20.

Family & Parenting Institute (2008) *Family & Parenting Institute: Research and Policy for the Real World*. Available at: http://www.familyandparenting.org/Filestore//Documents/aboutus/FPI_leaflet2.pdf (last accessed 25/09/2008).

Ferri E, Smith K (1996) *Parenting in the 1990s*. London: Family Policy Studies Centre, Joseph Rowntree Foundation.

Fisher D (2007) *Including New Fathers: A Guide for Maternity Professionals*. London: Fathers Direct. Available at: http://www.fatherhoodinstitute.org/index.php?id=2&cID=607 (last accessed 10/10/2008).

Geiger B (1996) *Fathers as Primary Caregivers*. Westport: Greenwood Press.

GenePool (2006) *Sickle Cell Anaemia*. Genetic Conditions Specialist Library, National Library for Health. Available at: http://www.library.nhs.uk/Genepool/ViewResource.aspx?resID=143175 (last accessed 24/07/08).

Hackel LS, Ruble DN (1992) Changes in the marital relationship after the first baby is born: predicting the impact of expectancy disconfirmation. *Journal of Personality and Social Psychology* 62 (6): 944–957.

Hall DMB, Elliman D (eds) (2006) *Health for All Children*, 4th Edition. Oxford, Oxford University Press.

Hansen TWR (2007) *Jaundice, Neonatal*. eMedicine. Available at: http://www.emedicine.com/ped/topic1061.htm (last accessed 17/10/2008).

Hoddinott P, Tappin D, Wright C (2008) Breastfeeding. Clinical review. *British Medical Journal* 336 (6749): 881–887.

Hogan M, Westcott C, Griffiths M (2005) Randomised, controlled trial of division of tongue-tie in infants with feeding problems. *Journal of Paediatrics and Child Health* 41 (5/6): 246–250.

Hooker E, Ball HL, Kelly PJ (2001) Sleeping like a baby: attitudes and experiences of bed sharing in northeast England. *Medical Anthropology* 19 (3): 203–222.

Knowles R, Griebsch I, Dezateux C, Brown J, Bull C, Wren C (2005) Newborn screening for congenital heart defects: a systematic review and cost-effectiveness analysis. *Health Technology Assessment* 9 (44): 1–152.

Kramer MS, Kakuma R (2002) Optimal duration of exclusive breastfeeding. *Cochrane Database of Systematic Reviews* 1. Art. No.: CD003517. DOI: 10.1002/14651858.CD003517.

Kreppner K (1988) Changes in parent ± child relationships with the birth of the second child. *Marriage and Family Review* 12 (3/4): 157–181.

Leonard BJ, Plotnikoff GA (2000) Awareness: the heart of cultural competence. *AACN Advanced Critical Care* 11(1): 51–59.

Lorenz L, Moyse K, Surguy H (2005) The benefits of baby massage. *Paediatric Nursing* 17(2): 15–18.

Maloni JA, Brezinski-Tomasi JE, Johnson LA (2001) Antepartum best rest: effect upon the family. *Journal of Obstetrics, Gynaecology and Neonatal Nursing* 30(2): 165–173.

McInnes RJ, Chambers JA (2008) Supporting breastfeeding mothers: qualitative synthesis. *Journal of Advanced Nursing* 62(4): 407–427.

Meleis AI (1997) *Theoretical Nursing: Development and Progress*. Philadelphia: Lippincott-Raven.

Mercer RT, Ferketich SL, May KA, DeJoesph J, Sollid D (1988) Further exploration of maternal and paternal fetal attachment. *Research in Nursing and Health* 11(2): 83–95.

Moore ER, Anderson GC, Bergman N (2007) Early skin-to-skin contact for mothers and their healthy newborn infants. *Cochrane Database of Systematic Reviews* 2. Art. No.: CD003519. DOI: 10.1002/14651858.CD003519.pub2.

Munro Cohen S (2006) Jaundice in the full term newborn. *Pediatric Nursing* 32(3): 202–208.

Muntaner C, Lynch J, Davey Smith G (2000) Social Capital and the third way in Public Health. *Critical Public Health* 10(2): 107–124.

National Institute for Health and Clinical Excellence (2005) *Division of Anky-loglossia (tongue-tie) for Breastfeeding*. London: NICE.

National Institute for Health and Clinical Excellence (2006) *Quick Reference Guide: Routine Post Natal Care of Women and their Babies*. NICE clinical guideline 37. London: NICE. Available at: http://www.nice.org.uk/nicemedia/pdf/CG37quickrefguide.pdf (last accessed 22/07/2008).

National Screening Committee (2000) *Second Report of the UK National Screening Committee*. London: DoH.

National Screening Committee (2003) *Criteria for Appraising the Viability, Effectiveness and Appropriateness of a Screening Programme*. London: NSC.

National Screening Committee (2008a) *Newborn and Infant Physical Examination: Standards and Competencies*. London: UK NSC.

National Screening Committee (2008b) *Guidelines for Newborn Blood Spot Sampling*. London: NSC.

National Screening Committee (2008c) *Standards and Guidelines for Newborn Blood Spot Screening*. London: NSC.

National Society for the Prevention of Cruelty to Children (2008) *Positive Parents make for Positive Families*. NSPCC. Available at: http://www.nspcc.org.uk/helpandadvice/publications/leaflets/positiveparents_wdf58146.pdf (last accessed 22/09/08).

Newman PR, Newman BM (1988) Parenthood and adult development. In: Palkovitz R, Sussman MB (eds). *Transitions to Parenthood*. New York: Haworth.

Partridge SE (1988) The parental self-concept: a theoretical exploration and practical application. *American Journal of Orthopsychiatry* 58(2): 281–287.

Prochaska JO, DiClemente CC (1982) Transtheoretical therapy: towards a more integrative model of change. *Psychotherapy Theory, Research, Practice* 19(3): 276–288.

Rogers CR (1953) *Client-centred Therapy. Its Current Practice, Implications and Theory*. Boston: Houghton Mifflin.

Rollnick S, Miller WR, Butler CC (2007) *Motivational Interviewing in Health Care: Helping Patients Change Behavior*. New York: Guildford Press.

Royal College of Midwives (2004) *Bed Sharing and Co-sleeping*. Position Statement No. 8. London: RCM.

Rubak S, Sandboek A, Lauritzen T, Christensen B (2005) Motivational Interviewing: a systematic review and meta-analysis. *British Journal of General Practice* 55(513): 305–312.

Rushforth B, Kini U (2003) Picture quiz: the genetics of cystic fibrosis. *Student British Medical Journal* 11: 405.

Sanders MR, Woolley MI (2005) The relationship between maternal self-efficacy and parenting practices: implications for parent training. *Child: Care, Health and Development* 31(1): 65–73.

Satir V (1990) *Peoplemaking*. London: Souvenir Press Ltd.

Seibert PS, Stridh-Igo P, Zimmerman CG (2002) A checklist to facilitate cultural awareness and sensitivity. *Journal of Medical Ethics* 28(3): 143–146.

Skinner H, Steinhauer P, Sitarenios G (2000) Family assessment measure (FAM) and process model of family functioning. *Journal of Family Therapy* 22(2): 190–210.

Stevenson DA, Dennery PA, Hintz SR (2001) Understanding newborn jaundice. *Journal of Perinatology* 21(S1): S21–S24.

Tammentie T, Paavilainen E, Astedt-Kurki P, Tarkka MT (2004) Family dynamics of postnatally depressed mothers – discrepancy between expectations and reality. *Journal of Clinical Nursing* 13(1): 65–74.

Taylor J, Daniel B (2000) The rhetoric vs. the reality in child care and protection: ideology and practice in working with fathers. *Journal of Advanced Nursing* 31(1): 12–19.

Townsend J, Wolke D, Hayes J (2004) Routine examination of the newborn: the EMREN study. Evaluation of an extension of the midwife role including a randomised controlled trial of appropriately trained midwives and paediatric senior house officers. *Health Technology Assessment* 8(14): 1–112.

UK Government (2004) *The Children's Act Chapter 31.* London: HMSO, TSO.

Watson Genna C (2007) *Supporting Sucking Skills in Breastfeeding Infants.* Sudbury, MA: Jones & Bartlett.

Wolke D, Dave S, Hayes J, Townsend J, Tomlin M (2002) Routine examination of the newborn and maternal satisfaction: a randomised controlled trial. *Archives of Disease in Childhood Fetal and Neonatal Edition* 86(3): 155–160.

World Health Organization (2002) *Global Strategy on Infant and Young Child Feeding.* Fifty Fifth World Health Assembly. Geneva: WHO.

Chapter 11
Sexual Health, Postnatal Care and Parenthood

Grace Edwards and Susie Gardiner

Introduction

> Methods and timing of resumption of contraception should be discussed within the first week of the birth.
>
> (NICE 2006a)

The postnatal period is the ideal time to address issues around sexual health and ensure that the woman and her partner are well informed about prevention of infection, family planning and risk taking. Too (2003) advocates that accurate, up-to-date information should be given regarding contraceptive methods, including their failure rates, health benefits and risks to enable the woman and her partner to make an informed decision. Indeed, this is reinforced by the National Institute for Health and Clinical Excellence (NICE) postnatal guidelines, which recommend that contraceptive issues should be discussed by the midwife within a week of the baby's birth and that good communication between healthcare professionals and women is essential. The guidelines also stress the need to support women who may have difficulty accessing contraceptive care. This includes providing contact details for expert contraceptive advice (NICE 2006a). Therefore, midwives have to have a sound knowledge of sexual health issues and contraception.

Sexual and reproductive health is not just the absence of disease or unintended pregnancy but also encompasses the positive aspect of relationships and sexuality. Improving sexual health therefore requires a holistic approach that incorporates the personal, social and emotional perspectives as well as the physical aspects of sex and sexuality. It is important that people have the life skills and values to make choices for themselves as well as have access to information and services for support and treatment.

Sexual and reproductive health can have a profound effect on individuals, communities and society: it is about overall good health care and pregnancy, the timing of which may, in turn, affect social outcomes, financial potential and future prospects. But there are also wider public health implications for poor sexual health. The Government's Public Health White Paper, 'Choosing Health: making healthier choices easier' (DoH 2004a) highlighted sexual health as a key priority for action, which is echoed in the White Paper, 'Our health our care our say' (DoH 2006a) and the National Health Service (NHS) Operating Framework (DoH 2007).

There is a clear relationship between sexual health problems, poverty and social exclusion (Hughes *et al.* 2006). Poor sexual health can be severely debilitating and some sexually transmitted infections (STIs), if left untreated, can have extremely serious consequences such as the development of pelvic inflammatory disease, chronic abdominal pain, infertility and ectopic pregnancy. Thus, pregnancy and the postnatal period are ideal times to discuss prevention and treatment.

Sexual health today

The Independent Advisory Group on Sexual Health and HIV recently commissioned the Medical Foundation for AIDS and Sexual Health to review the 2001 Sexual Health Strategy (DoH 2001) and make recommendations for further action. The report, 'Progress and Priorities – Working Together for High Quality Sexual Health' (MedFASH 2008), comments on the impact that the Strategy has had since 2001, and identified five key strategic areas for action:

- Prioritising sexual health as a key public health issue and sustaining high-level leadership at local, regional and national levels
- Building strategic partnerships
- Improved commissioning for sexual health
- Investing more in prevention
- Improved delivery of sexual health services

Although from a midwifery point of view, the focus is on antenatal screening, it is equally important that contraception and sexual health care are discussed with women post-natally. Indeed, the report highlights the need for midwives to be part of an overall, comprehensive sexual health provision, particularly for most at-risk and young people aged under 18 years.

Sexual health has got worse in the United Kingdom over recent years, with large increases in many STIs. The diagnosis of chlamydia in genitourinary medicine (GUM) clinics has increased by 166% (from 1997 to 2006), and gonorrhoea by over 46% in the same time period (to 19 007 diagnoses) (HPA 2008a). There has also been an increase in the incidence of HIV, from 2800 cases diagnosed in 1997 to nearly 6500 in 2007 (HPA 2008b).

It is useful for midwives to have some knowledge about the aetiology and prevalence of some of the more common STIs.

Chlamydia

A common example of an infection where many people are unaware that they are infected is chlamydia. Levels of infection in the United Kingdom have more than doubled over the past 10 years, particularly in teenagers. In 2007, genital chlamydial infection remained the most common STI diagnosed in GUM clinics in the United Kingdom. Chlamydia is a bacterial infection that can be treated and cured orally with antibiotics; however, it has no symptoms in at least 70% of women and 50% of men (HPA 2008a). In 2007, the National Chlamydia Screening Programme performed 270 729 screens for young people aged 15–24 years. Of these, 9.5% young women and 8.4% young men tested positive for the infection.

HIV and AIDS

The number of people with HIV is also worrying. By the end of 2006, there were an estimated 73 000 people living with HIV in the United Kingdom, of which an estimated 21 600 people were unaware they had become infected. The prevalence of HIV in pregnant women living outside of London has increased 8-fold between 1997 and 2006 (HPA 2008a). The good news is that rates of detection are high in pregnant women, with 90% HIV-infected women diagnosed prior to delivery. Although most midwives are familiar with dealing with women with HIV, it is worth revisiting how the infection is transmitted.

The human immunodeficiency virus (HIV) that causes AIDS is transmitted through body fluids, in particular blood, semen, vaginal secretions and breast milk. You can become infected with HIV through the following:

- Unprotected sexual intercourse with an infected partner
- Sharing needles when injecting or other use of contaminated injection or other skin piercing equipment

- Blood and blood products, for example, infected transfusions and organ tissue transplants
- Transmission from infected mother to child in the womb or at birth and breastfeeding

In the United Kingdom, there has also been an increase in the number of people who have become infected through heterosexual partners, suggesting that messages on HIV and STIs are being ignored (HPA 2005). According to the 2007 epidemiological data published by the Health Protection Agency (2008a), approximately 1 in every 440 pregnant women in the United Kingdom was HIV-infected. Most cases were identified in women who themselves were born in high prevalence regions, particularly sub-Saharan Africa and Central America and the Caribbean. However, the prevalence of HIV among women born in the United Kingdom continues to rise slowly.

There is a risk that HIV-positive mothers may transmit HIV to their babies through breastfeeding. Therefore, for babies born to HIV-positive mothers, the risk of passing on HIV through breastfeeding must be balanced against the risk of infection and death if they are not breastfed. In the United Kingdom, women who are HIV positive are advised not to breastfeed their babies as the risk of HIV transmission is greater than the risks of artificial feeding (Unicef UK 2006).

Good practice point

Discuss methods of feeding with women who are HIV positive in the ante-natal period. Practices are different in sub-Sahara countries.

Other sexually transmitted infections

Over the past 10 years, there has been a 46% increase in the number of new cases of gonorrhoea reported (HPA 2008a). Young people in the United Kingdom are disproportionately affected by gonorrhoea and also chlamydia (as discussed earlier) and genital warts. Rates of diagnoses continued to increase among young people in 2007 (50% of all diagnoses are made for young people aged 16–24 years), with the highest rates of gonorrhoea diseases seen among young men aged 20–24 years (HPA 2008a).

Diagnoses of syphilis rose by a staggering 1607% from 1997 to 2006, although this is driven partly by outbreaks such as those found in Manchester and London. Syphilis is still relatively uncommon, with 2766 diagnoses in 2006. However, it is especially significant for pregnant women where infection can cause miscarriage, still birth or fetal abnormality.

The most commonly diagnosed viral STI is genital warts. From 1997 to 2006, new diagnoses of genital warts rose by 22% to 83 745 (HPA 2008a). Again the highest rates were seen in younger age groups, men aged 20–24 and worryingly young women aged 16–19. The prevalence of genital warts is likely to be vastly underestimated as figures are only available for people who report for treatment. Similar trends are apparent for genital herpes.

Recent UK trends in sexual activity and behaviours

Whilst the introduction of the National Chlamydia Screening Programme and encouragement for people to access STI testing and treatment services may have contributed to this increase in diagnoses, studies have shown a change in patterns of sexual behaviour in the United Kingdom.

The recent and continued increase in the diagnoses of new episodes of STIs in the United Kingdom and the high rates of teenage conceptions are an indication of an increase in sexual risk-taking behaviour amongst many population groups (Fenton & Hughes 2003).

Between 1990 and 2000, the age at first intercourse dropped from 17 years to 16 years. In 2000, over a quarter (26%) of 16- to 19-year-old females were under 16 years when they first had sexual intercourse (young people who are socially disadvantaged are more likely to have sex at less than 16 years). Using a measurement for preparedness for sexual activity (reasons for sexual intercourse and use of a reliable method of contraception), less than half of those having first intercourse before the age of 16 were defined as being prepared (Johnson *et al*. 2001).

One of the aims of the teenage pregnancy strategy is to reduce the number of subsequent pregnancies in teenagers. However, it is not only teenagers who may need support in family spacing. In order to be able to address this, midwives need to understand some of the factors that may affect women in controlling their fertility. Ellis *et al*. (2003) found that sexual behaviour may be influenced by a number of factors including the following:

- Low self-esteem
- Lack of skills, for example, how to use a condom
- Lack of negotiation skills, for example, how to say 'No' to sex without a condom
- Lack of knowledge about the risks of different sexual behaviours
- Availability of resources – contraceptives and access to services
- Peer pressure

- Attitudes and the stigmatisation of sexual health in society, which may affect people's willingness to access services

These factors may still be relevant in the postnatal period.

Good practice point

Sexual health and contraception should be discussed in the antenatal period.

In addition to the documented changes in patterns of sexual behaviours and attitudes in the United Kingdom, levels of awareness about STIs are also poor in the United Kingdom. A recently commissioned survey that sought views from over 2000 people over the age of 15 (National AIDS Trust 2006) found that many of those who participated were not aware that HIV could be transmitted from one person to another through unprotected sex. Even more alarmingly, 15% of those surveyed said that they would never or rarely use a condom the first time they had sex with a new partner, with only 10% prepared to undergo testing for HIV before stopping using a condom in a new relationship.

Some midwives may feel embarrassed about addressing issues such as lack of knowledge of women around safe sex, but this is an important part of our practice. By using strategies such as brief intervention techniques, messages can be portrayed in an informative, non-judgemental way. Brief intervention strategies have been used for sometime in supporting health behavioural changes and have proven to be effective, particularly in the management of individuals with hazardous and harmful drinking and smoking cessation. The NICE guidelines for smoking cessation (NICE 2006c) describe a simple brief intervention that typically takes between 5 and 10 minutes and may include one or more of the following:

- Simple opportunistic advice to stop
- An assessment of the patient's commitment to quit
- An offer of pharmacotherapy and/or behavioural support
- Provision of self-help material and referral to more intensive support such as the NHS Stop Smoking Services

If this simple model was related to sexual health and contraceptive advice, it may include the following:

- Simple advice on STIs and their prevention
- A simple assessment of the client's knowledge around sexual health and contraception

- Referral to appropriate contraceptive and sexual health services
- Provision of leaflets and contact numbers for community support

---

Good practice point

Brief interventions work!! Learn the technique to apply to all health promotion issues.

The cost of poor sexual health

The Health Protection Agency estimates that the yearly costs of treating STIs in the United Kingdom is over £700 million, and this figure does not take into account the amount of money invested in treating illness that results as a consequence of an undiagnosed infection for example, ectopic pregnancy and infertility.

The message is clear – prevention is better than cure. Prevention not only reduces the burden of ill health to the community but also to the NHS and the system. In addition to the above, from a common sense health protection perspective, the fewer infected people there are, the smaller the risk of onward transmission to others.

In 2005, research undertaken for the Family Planning Association by Armstrong and Donaldson estimated that there are big savings to be made by investing in contraception. This research also suggested that the figure could be increased significantly even further by revising the current supply of NHS contraceptive methods to better reflect what women prefer, thus potentially leading to a reduction in the number of unplanned pregnancies and abortions. They estimated that this could bring about an additional cost saving of up to £1 billion over 15 years (Armstrong & Donaldson 2005).

Government policy and guidance

NICE guidance – under-18 conceptions and STIs

This guidance recommends that midwives and health visitors who provide antenatal, postnatal and child development care should do the following:

- Regularly visit vulnerable women aged under 18 who are pregnant or who are already mothers.

- Discuss with them and their partner (where appropriate) how to prevent or get tested for STIs and how to prevent unwanted pregnancies. The discussion should cover

  – all methods of reversible contraception, including long-acting reversible contraception (LARC) (in line with NICE clinical guideline 30), and how to get and use emergency contraception;
  – health promotion advice, in line with NICE guidance on postnatal care (NICE clinical guideline 37);
  – opportunities for returning to education, training and employment in the future.

- Provide supporting information in an appropriate format.
- Where appropriate, refer the young woman to the relevant agencies, including services concerned with reintegration into education and work.

This enhanced care should particularly target young women from disadvantaged backgrounds, those in or leaving care and those with a low educational attainment.

These recommendations can also be utilised for other vulnerable groups.

NICE guidance – LARC

In October 2005, NICE published guidance on LARC (NICE 2005) that highlighted the need for informed healthcare professionals to enable women to make decisions about their reproductive health. It also stressed the importance of clear commissioning pathways that can take advantage of the cost-effectiveness of LARC when compared to other contraceptive methods. The guidance aims to assist both clinicians and patients in making decisions about the most appropriate treatment. Whilst it is not expected that midwives are able to administer LARC methods, it is key that they are able to discuss these methods and signpost women to suitable services.

LARC is taken up by an estimated 10% of women aged under 50 (although 45% would use this method if offered) (Armstrong & Donaldson 2005). Oral contraceptives and male condoms are the most commonly used methods of contraception, with uptake of 25 and 22% respectively (ONS 2006). Uptake of LARC is fairly low when compared with other contraceptive methods (NICE 2006b).

It is vital that midwives are up to date with recommendations such as those contained within the NICE guidance. Midwives are well placed to discuss future contraceptive use, and the option of using LARC may be of particular benefit to a woman who may have more difficulty in complying with user-dependent contraceptives such as the contraceptive pill. The guidelines do highlight, however, that particularly for young women and those who are considered to be at greater risk of infection, health professionals need to highlight that LARC does not provide protection against STIs and that barrier methods, for example, the condom, should still be used in addition to LARC.

In addition to the NICE guidance, the National Service Framework for Children, *Young People and Maternity Services* (DoH 2004b) recommends that support in the community is available for vulnerable groups such as teenage parents, with relevant agencies such as Connexions, including the provision of contraceptive advice and treatment. It is still important to remember that over a quarter of births in young women aged 17 and 18 are second pregnancies. Although some of these will be planned, many are not. Good-quality contraceptive advice and treatment are essential to ensure that young women are able to prevent subsequent pregnancies if they wish to (DoH 2004b; ONS 2006).

Good practice point

Visit the NICE web site regularly at nice.org.uk to ensure that you have the latest evidence-based guidance on which to base your practice.

Chlamydia screening programme

The National Chlamydia Screening Programme was set up in 2003 and aims to

- prevent and control chlamydia through early detection and treatment of asymptomatic infection;
- reduce onward transmission to sexual partners;
- prevent the consequences of untreated infection.

The programme has been fully operational across the country since April 2007 and aims to achieve its goals through a multifaceted, evidence-based and cost-effective programme. Local areas each have a screening programme co-ordinator, who ensures that all sexually active young men and women aged 15–24 years are aware of chlamydia and its effects as well as of increasing access to services that provide screening, prevention and treatment. This service has a community focus and concentrates on opportunistic screening of asymptomatic sexually active men and women under the age of 25 who would not normally access, or be offered a chlamydia test, and focuses on screening in non-traditional sites such as youth services, military bases, universities, contraception services, and primary care (DoH 2008).

Teenage pregnancy strategy

In addition to the 1999 'Teenage Pregnancy Strategy' (DoH 1999), the more recent 'Accelerating the Strategy to 2010' (DfES 2006) identified the following key themes to be developed and strengthened:

- Active engagement of all key delivery partners
- A strong senior champion
- Availability of well-publicised, young people-centred contraceptive and sexual health advice service with a strong remit to undertake health promotion work
- High priority given to personal, social and health education (PSHE) in schools
- Strong focus on targeted interventions with young people at greatest risk, in particular looked after children
- Workforce training: availability and take-up of sex and relationship education (SRE) training
- Well-resourced youth service with a clear focus on addressing key social issues

Midwifery is a key partner and is well placed to advise and support the local strategies, including both appropriate provision for teenage mothers and advice and/or signposting to sexual health services delivered in a non-judgemental and supportive environment. The Teenage Pregnancy Strategy links to a number of other policy drivers, some of which are listed below.

New contraception funding

In 2008, the Department of Health (2008), announced £26.8 million new funding for contraception, identifying contraception as a priority for action. The funding aims to encourage innovative programmes to improve access to contraception and will provide an information campaign on contraceptive choices for young people.

Other policies

In addition to all of the above, which specifically refer to improving sexual health, there are broader policy documents that also impact on attempts to improve sexual health and they include *Every Child Matters: Change for Children* (DfES 2004) – the key policy document for improving outcomes for children and young people, which focuses on being healthy, staying safe, enjoying and achieving, making a positive contribution and achieving economic well-being; *Our Health, Our Care, Our Say* (DoH 2006a) – the key policy document for the provision of integrated services in the community, which refers explicitly to sexual health services; and *Creating a Patient-led NHS: Delivering the NHS Improvement Plan* (DoH 2005) – which focuses on encouraging an informed choice and on NHS organisations becoming more focused and better at understanding the needs of their patients and commissioning services that more effectively meet the needs of the local population.

Whilst a national commitment to improving sexual health in key policy documents is welcomed, it is important that these policies are a real lever for change at the local level, which, in turn, will lead to improvements in sexual health outcomes for our populations.

Vulnerable groups

The 'Independent Enquiry into Health Inequalities in Health' report (Acheson 1998) recognised the gap that exists between the advantaged and disadvantaged groups in society, and recommended that local solutions should be sought to reduce these inequalities. In particular, it emphasised the need for targeted prevention and support for vulnerable groups. We have highlighted two groups for this purpose where health inequalities exist, as below.

Teenage parents

The United Kingdom still has one of the highest rates of teenage pregnancy in Western Europe. Although some progress has been made since the baseline statistics of 1998 (by 2006, the national teenage conception rate had decreased from 46.6 to 40.6 per 1000: ONS 2008), there were 39 170 under-18 conceptions in 2006. Of these, 49% resulted in abortion.

Teenage pregnancy is often associated with poor health and negative social outcomes for both the mother and child. Although teenage pregnancy is not biologically harmful, young mothers are more likely to have adverse outcomes socially, economically and in terms of health status (HDA 1999). Some research indicates that young people who have been disadvantaged in childhood and/or have grown up in poverty and have low expectations in life are more likely to become teenage parents (Botting *et al.* 1998; Gillham 1997). Difficulties in young people's lives such as poor family relationships, low self-esteem and dislike of school also contribute to young people's risk (DfES DH 2007). The children are less likely to be breast-fed, more likely to live in poverty and more likely to become teenage parents themselves (Botting *et al.* 1998).

The Teenage Pregnancy Strategy has highlighted the following risk factors which increase the likelihood of teenage pregnancy.

- Risky behaviours:
  - Early onset of sexual activity
  - Poor contraceptive use
  - A mental health problem, a conduct disorder and/or involvement in crime
  - Alcohol and substance misuse
  - Already a teenage mother or had an abortion.

- Education-related factors:
  - Low education attainment or no qualifications
  - Disengagement from school.

- Family/background:
  - Living in care
  - Daughter of a teenage mother
  - Daughter of a mother who has low educational aspirations for them
  - Belonging to a particular ethnic group (in the 2001 census, 'mixed White', 'Black Caribbean', 'other Black' and 'White British' were over-represented among teenage mothers)

A recent government document *Multi-agency Working to Support Pregnant Teenagers* (DfES 2007) highlights the importance of midwifery services adopting a partnership model of working with other agencies to meet the often complex needs of pregnant teenagers and new teenage mothers. Working in partnership provides the best joined up service for all women and may save midwifery time by referring women to agencies best equipped to support them, for example, Connexions (DfES 2007).

Good practice point

What is the teenage pregnancy rate in your area?
How does it compare with other local areas?
How does it fit into the national picture?
What can you do to support the teenage pregnancy strategy?

Women living in deprived areas/with low educational achievement

It is well documented that those living in deprivation are more likely to experience lower levels of education attainment. A recent study by Rutherford *et al.* (2006) examined whether there are links between low levels of literacy and sexual behaviour and knowledge. Their study concluded that there is a link and moreover that those in the lower literacy group were

- significantly more likely to have been under 16 years of age the first time they had sex;
- significantly less likely to know when the most fertile time is during the menstrual cycle;
- significantly less likely to be able to identify STIs;
- significantly less likely to be aware that infections can be transmitted through both oral and anal sex;
- more likely to have difficulties understanding health literature distributed in clinics.

A summary fact sheet on sexual health from the Department of Health (DoH 2006b) concurred with this evidence and stated that STIs disproportionately affect young people and that STIs are more prevalent in deprived areas with poor educational attainment and low aspiration.

Women suffering domestic violence

One in four women will suffer domestic abuse in their lives and 30% of cases of domestic violence start during pregnancy. This is a shocking statistic as most people cannot believe that a partner could be violent towards a pregnant woman. Domestic abuse occurs across the whole of society, regardless of race, ethnicity and religion, age, class and income.

Pregnancy and the postnatal period may form a window of opportunity for women to disclose domestic abuse to a midwife and it is important that midwives can handle disclosure sensitively and efficiently. The NICE postnatal guidelines (DoH 2006a) recommend that all healthcare professionals should be aware of the risks, signs and symptoms of domestic abuse and know who to contact for advice and management, following guidance from the Department of Health. For in-depth information on dealing with domestic abuse, please see *Responding to Domestic Abuse: a Handbook for Health Professionals* (Department of Health 2006c). Available from www.dh.gov.uk

> **Good practice point**
>
> Is routine enquiry in place in your area of work?
> Are you familiar with your domestic abuse guidelines?
> Do you know where to find the referral pathway?

Midwifery and targeted actions

Research by Dwyer (2001) found that pregnant women were largely unaware of the dangers associated with STIs during pregnancy. She found that 91% of couples rarely or never used condoms, either before or during pregnancy despite the fact that 95% of women were unaware of their partner's infection status. Over half of the women sampled were ignorant about the effect of STIs on their pregnancy. Over one quarter of the women (27%) had multiple partners during their pregnancy.

We have already discussed the National Chlamydia Screening Programme and how the programme offers opportunistic screening to under-25s in community settings and aims to pick up those asymptomatic young people and their partners who otherwise would not have come forward for testing. There has been some discussion nationally around whether or not chlamydia screening for the under-25s should become a standard screen offered to pregnant women as chlamydia infection can be transmitted from mother to child. Screening may be an effective mechanism for reducing this transmission as some treatments for chlamydia can be prescribed during pregnancy.

There are many reasons why midwives do not discuss safer sex during pregnancy. It may be that midwives are unsure of their own knowledge base around sexual health, are anxious about upsetting women or their partners, or they may be embarrassed about discussing sexual health issues. However, the fact that women are pregnant means that they have had unprotected sex and although this does not mean that they have had unsafe sex, there are ideal opportunities to deliver sexual health promotion messages during pregnancy and post-natally. Key times for discussion include booking, screening visits, whether the midwife is aware of a change of partner and during the postnatal period.

Midwives are clinicians key to informing and supporting women around good sexual health. It is important that we see this as part of our public health role, intrinsic to our clinical role and do not see it as someone else's job, or a golden opportunity will be missed.

> ## Key implications for midwifery practice
>
> Who is your PCT lead for sexual health?
> Encourage condom use in women with a new or casual partner.
> Pregnancy and the postnatal period are windows of opportunity to influence future sexual health.
> Do you know where your local GUM clinic is? What advice and treatment is offered?
> Is there a Brook clinic or another young person's sexual health service in your area? Do you know how to refer young women?
> Who is your local teenage pregnancy coordinator?
> Get involved with your local chlamydia screening programme.
> Do you have access to condom distribution?
> Are there opportunities for midwives to access additional training around family planning and sexual health?
> What information is available both locally and nationally for women who disclose domestic abuse?
> Have you accessed brief intervention training?

References

Acheson D (1998) *Independent Inquiry into Inequalities in Health*. London: The Stationery Office.

Armstrong N and Donaldson C (2005) *The Economics of Sexual Health*. London: Findings FPA.

Botting B, Rosato M, Wood R (1998) *Teenage Mothers and the Health of their Children*, Population Trends, 93; Autumn. London: ONS.

Department for Education and Skills (2004) *Every Child Matters: Change for Children*. London: DfES.

Department for Education and Skills (2006) *Accelerating the Strategy to 2010*. London: DfES.

Department for Education and Skills (2007) *Multi-agency Working to Support Pregnant Teenagers: A Midwifery Guide to Partnership Working with Connexions and Other Agencies*. London: DfES and DH.

Department of Health (1999) *Teenage Pregnancy: A Social Exclusion Unit Report*. London: DoH.

Department of Health (2001) *The National Strategy for Sexual Health and HIV*. London: DoH.

Department of Health (2004a) *Choosing Health White Paper*. London: DoH.

Department of Health (2004b) *National Service Framework for Children, Young People and Maternity Services*. London: DoH.

Department of Health (2005) *Creating a Patient-led NHS: Delivering the NHS Improvement Plan*. London: DoH.

Department of Health (2006a) *Our Health, Our Care, Our Say: Making it Happen*. London: DoH.

Department of Health (2006b) *Fact Sheet on Sexual Health*. London: DoH.

Department of Health (2006c) *Responding to Domestic Abuse: A Handbook for Health Professionals*. London: DoH.

Department of Health (2007) *The NHS in England: The Operating Framework for 2008–2009*.

Department of Health (2008) *Annual Report of the National Chlamydia Screening Programme in England 2007/08*. Chlamydiascreening.nhs.uk/ps/aboutindex.html (accessed August 2008)

Dwyer JM (2001) High-risk sexual behaviours and genital infections during pregnancy. *International Nurse Reviewer* 48 (4): 233–240.

Ellis S, Barnett-Page, E, Morgan, A (2003) *HIV Prevention: A Review of Reviews Assessing the Effectiveness of Interventions to Reduce the Risk of Sexual Transmission*. London: Health Development Agency.

Fenton KA, Hughes G (2003) Sexual behaviour in Britain: why sexually transmitted infections are common. *Clinical Medicine: Journal of the Royal College of Physicians* 3 (3) 84–92.

Health Development Agency (1999) *Reducing the Rate of Teenage Conceptions: An International Review of the Evidence*. Available from: www.nice.org.uk/ (accessed 29 August 2008).

Health Protection Agency (2005) *HIV and other Sexually Transmitted Infections in the UK*. London: HPA.

Health Protection Agency (2008a) *Epidemiological Data – Sexually Transmitted Infections [Online]*. Available from: www.hpa.org.uk/infections/topics_az/hiv_and_sti/epidemiology/sti_data.htm (accessed 29/08/2008).

Health Protection Agency and Health Protection Scotland (2008b) (Unpublished) *New HIV Diagnoses Surveillance Tables*. Available from: www.hpa.org.uk/infections/topics_az/hiv_and_sti/hiv/epidemiology/files (accessed 29/08/2008).

Hughes S, Moeller H, Cook P, Ashraf A, Tocque K, Bellis M (2006) *Sexual and Reproductive Health Indicators for the North Wes*. Liverpool: Centre for Public Health.

Gillham B (1997) *The Facts about Teenage Pregnancies* London: Cassell.

Johnson AM, Mercer CH, Erens B, *et al.* (2001) Sexual behaviour in Britain: partnerships, practices, and HIV risk behaviours. *Lancet* 358 (9296): 1835–1842.

MedFASH (Medical Foundation for AIDS and Sexual Health) (2008) *Progress and Priorities – Working Together for High Quality Sexual Health*. London: MedFASH.

National AIDS Trust (2006) Public lack of knowledge of HIV. *The Pharmaceutical Journal* 276: 559.

National Institute for Health and Clinical Excellence (2005) *Long-acting Reversible Contraception: The Effective and Appropriate Use of Long-acting Reversible Contraception*. London: NICE.

National Institute for Health and Clinical Excellence (2006a) *Routine Postnatal Care of Women and their Babies*. London: NICE.

National Institute for Health and Clinical Excellence (2006b) *Preventing Sexually Transmitted Infections and Reducing Under-18 Conceptions Draft Guidance for Consultation*. London: NICE.

National Institute for Health and Clinical Excellence (2006c) *Brief Interventions and Referral for Smoking Cessation: Guidance*.

Office of National Statistics (2006) *Contraception and Sexual Health 2004–2005*. London: Office for National Statistics.

Office for National Statistics (2008) *Under 18 Conceptions Data for Top-tier Local Authorities (LAD1), 1998–2006*. London: Office for National Statistics and the Teenage Pregnancy Unit.

Rutherford J, Holman R, MacDonald J, *et al.* (2006) Low Literacy: a hidden problem in family planning clinics. *Journal of Family Planning and Reproductive Health Care* 32 (4): 235–240.

Too S-K (2003) Breastfeeding and contraception. *British Journal of Midwifery* 11 (2): 88–93.

Unicef UK (2006) *Unicef Policy on Infant Feeding*. http://www.unicef.org.uk/unicefuk/policies/policy_detail (accessed August 2008).

Further reading

Department of Health (2005) *Responding to Domestic Abuse: A Handbook for Health Professionals*. London: Department of Health. Available from: www.dh.gov.uk (accessed 29 August 2008).

NICE (2007a) *Routine Postnatal Care of Women and their Babies*, Clinical guideline 37. London: National Collaborating Centre for Primary Care.

NICE (2007b) *One to One Interventions to Reduce the Transmission of Sexually Transmitted Infections (STIs) Including HIV, and to Reduce the Rate of Under 18 Conceptions, Especially Among Vulnerable and at Risk Groups*, Public Health Intervention Guidance 3. London: NICE.

Index

Note: page numbers in *italics* refer to figures, and those in **bold** to tables or boxes.